Galveston Diet Cookbook For Beginners

2000 Days of Delicious and Wholesome Hormone-Balancing and Anti-Inflammatory Recipes for Effective Weight Loss and Optimal Menopausal Health

Amanda K. Sanders

Table of Contents

Introduction to the Galveston Diet

An Overview of the Galveston Diet

The Galveston Diet is a unique and tailored approach to nutrition and wellness, specifically designed to cater to the needs of women in midlife. Unlike many generic diet plans, the Galveston Diet focuses on the intricate relationship between diet, hormones, and inflammation. The main objectives of this approach are to support weight loss, regulate hormones, and decrease inflammation, providing a comprehensive approach to health that goes beyond simply counting calories.

The Galveston Diet emphasizes nutrient-dense, anti-inflammatory foods while discouraging the consumption of processed carbohydrates and sugars. By emphasizing the consumption of whole, unprocessed foods, this diet promotes stable blood sugar levels, contributing to weight management and lowering the risk of chronic diseases. The Galveston Diet also includes intermittent fasting, known for its positive effects on metabolic health, cellular repair, and insulin sensitivity.

The Galveston Diet offers a wide range of benefits. Regarding weight loss, the main focus is on developing a long-lasting, healthy relationship with food that avoids the pitfalls of restrictive dieting. Proper hormone balance can be achieved by making specific dietary choices promoting endocrine health. These choices can help address common issues such as insulin resistance and estrogen dominance that often affect women in midlife. Ultimately, the diet's anti-inflammatory properties can effectively reduce chronic inflammation, a critical factor in various age-related diseases. This, in turn, supports overall health and vitality.

Scientific Basis

The science behind the Galveston Diet is based on an in-depth understanding of how specific foods and eating habits impact our bodies at a biochemical level. An essential aspect of this diet is its emphasis on anti-inflammatory foods. Chronic inflammation has been associated with various health issues, such as heart disease, diabetes, and autoimmune conditions. The Galveston diet emphasizes consuming foods packed with antioxidants, omega-3 fatty acids, and phytonutrients. This dietary approach aims to reduce inflammation and provide protection against various diseases.

Intermittent fasting is a fundamental aspect of the Galveston Diet. This eating pattern involves alternating between periods of eating and fasting, which has been demonstrated to positively affect metabolic health, brain function, and lifespan. Fasting periods enable the body to undergo autophagy, a natural process that eliminates and repairs damaged cells, enhancing cellular function and resilience.

The Galveston Diet requires reducing processed carbohydrates. Consuming processed carbohydrates and sugars can result in fluctuations in blood sugar and insulin levels, contributing to weight gain and raising the risk of developing metabolic disorders. By excluding certain foods, the diet aims to stabilize blood sugar levels, improve insulin sensitivity, and facilitate weight loss.

Scientific studies have consistently demonstrated that diets that prioritize whole, unprocessed foods and limit refined carbohydrates can significantly improve one's health. The Galveston Diet incorporates these findings into a practical, user-friendly plan that promotes long-term health and well-being.

Who Should Read This Book

"Galveston Diet Cookbook for Beginners" is perfect for individuals seeking to enhance their well-being with a proven, comprehensive approach to nutrition. However, it is particularly helpful for middle-aged women experiencing hormonal changes linked to perimenopause and menopause.

During midlife, women often encounter specific challenges, including weight gain, particularly around the midsection, hormonal fluctuations, and increased inflammation. These changes may result in various symptoms, such as fatigue, mood swings, and a higher risk of chronic diseases. The Galveston diet directly addresses these concerns by emphasizing foods and practices that promote hormonal health, reduce inflammation, and facilitate sustainable weight loss.

If you are facing challenges with weight gain, hormonal imbalance, or seeking a healthier eating approach, this book is tailored to your needs. It offers practical guidance, mouthwatering recipes, and a thorough understanding of how the Galveston Diet can assist you in reaching your health objectives. This cookbook is a valuable resource for those looking to adopt a healthier eating approach that caters to their body's requirements during midlife and beyond. It aims to help you feel your absolute best and lead a life of optimal health.

Chapter 1

Nutritional Guidelines and Food Lists

Core Nutritional Principles

The Galveston Diet is designed to promote optimal health by focusing on a well-balanced mix of macronutrients, emphasizing healthy fats, lean proteins, and fiber-rich carbohydrates. Here is a comprehensive review of the fundamental nutritional principles of the diet:

1. Healthy Fats:

- **Recommended Daily Intake:** 30-40% of total daily calories

- **Sources:** Avocados, nuts, seeds, olive oil, fatty fish (like salmon and mackerel), and coconut oil

- **Benefits:** Consuming healthy fats is essential for maintaining hormone production, supporting brain health, and minimizing inflammation. They offer a consistent energy supply and contribute to a sense of satiety.

2. Lean Proteins:

- **Recommended Daily Intake:** 25-35% of total daily calories

- **Sources:** Poultry, fish, lean cuts of beef, eggs, tofu, legumes, and low-fat dairy products

- **Benefits:** Protein is crucial in muscle repair and growth, immune function, and maintaining a healthy metabolism. It also contributes to hormone balance and overall health support.

3. Fiber-Rich Carbohydrates:

- **Recommended Daily Intake:** 25-30% of total daily calories

- **Sources:** Vegetables, fruits, whole grains, legumes, and seeds

- **Benefits:** Fiber aids digestion, maintains stable blood sugar levels, and supports a healthy gut microbiome. Additionally, it is linked to a lower likelihood of developing chronic conditions like heart disease and diabetes.

4. The Role of Fiber:

- The Galveston diet particularly emphasizes fiber for its many health benefits. It aids in hunger management, promotes digestive well-being, and supports the body's detoxification processes. High-fiber foods are packed with essential nutrients and are usually lower in calories, making them an excellent choice for managing weight.

Allowed and Restricted Foods

Having a clear understanding of the foods to include and those to avoid is essential for effectively following the Galveston Diet. Here is a comprehensive breakdown of the foods that are permitted and those that are not, along with explanations of their benefits or drawbacks:

1. Recommended Foods:

- **Vegetables:** Leafy greens, broccoli, cauliflower, bell peppers, and Brussels sprouts. These foods contain a rich array of vitamins, minerals, and antioxidants that reduce inflammation and promote overall well-being.

- **Fruits:** Berries, apples, pears, and citrus fruits. These fruits offer a great balance of fiber and antioxidants, with a lower sugar content compared to other fruits.

- **Healthy Fats:** Avocados, olive oil, nuts, seeds, and fatty fish. These fats benefit heart health, help reduce inflammation, and contain essential fatty acids.

- **Lean Proteins:** Chicken, turkey, fish, eggs, tofu, and legumes. These proteins are rich in essential nutrients and low in unhealthy fats.

- **Whole Grains:** Quinoa, brown rice, oats, and barley. Whole grains offer a range of benefits, including complex carbohydrates, fiber, and essential nutrients.

- **Legumes:** include lentils, chickpeas, black beans, and kidney beans. These are excellent sources of plant-based protein and fiber.

2. Foods Allowed in Moderation:

- **Dairy:** Greek yogurt, cottage cheese, and hard cheeses. Although dairy products can provide essential nutrients like calcium and protein, they should be consumed in moderation because they may have inflammatory effects.

- **Whole Grains:** Whole grains can be a valuable addition to a balanced diet, but it's critical to be mindful of portion sizes to maintain a healthy carbohydrate intake.

- **Fruits with Higher Sugar Content:** Bananas, grapes, and mangoes are among fruits with a higher sugar content. Consuming these in moderation is advisable to prevent sudden increases in blood sugar levels.

3. Foods to Avoid:

- **Processed Carbohydrates:** Includes white bread, pastries, and sugary cereals. These foods can lead to sudden increases in blood sugar levels and contribute to weight gain and inflammation.

- **Sugary beverages:** These include sodas, energy drinks, and sweetened coffees. The high sugar content in these drinks can contribute to insulin resistance and metabolic issues.

- **Trans Fats:** Also known as bad fat, trans fat is commonly found in fried foods, margarine, and commercially baked goods. They are strongly inflammatory and can significantly raise the risk of developing chronic diseases.

- **Processed Meats:** Sausages, hot dogs, and deli meats frequently include unhealthy fats, additives, and preservatives that can negatively affect health.

- **Excessive Alcohol:** Although moderate alcohol consumption may be acceptable, consuming too much can result in weight gain, hormonal imbalances, and heightened inflammation.

Supplement Recommendations

Along with a well-rounded diet, incorporating specific supplements can further optimize the benefits of the Galveston Diet by supplying vital nutrients that may be deficient:

1.Omega-3 Fatty Acids:

- **Source:** Fish oil or algae-based supplements

- **Benefits:** Omega-3s have been shown to have positive effects on inflammation, heart and brain health, as well as mood and hormone balance.

2. Vitamin D:

- **Source:** Supplements containing Vitamin D3

- **Benefits:** Vitamin D is essential for maintaining strong bones, supporting a healthy immune system, and regulating mood. This is especially important for women during midlife.

3. Magnesium:

- **Source:** Supplements containing magnesium citrate or glycinate

- **Benefits:** Magnesium has positive effects on muscle and nerve function, blood sugar regulation, and sleep quality.

4. Probiotics:

- **Source:** Probiotic supplements with diverse strains

- **Benefits:** Probiotics are crucial for maintaining a healthy gut microbiome, which is vital for digestion, immune function, and inflammation reduction.

5. Fiber Supplements:

- **Source:** Supplements containing psyllium husk, inulin, or acacia fiber

- **Benefits:** These can assist in maintaining a healthy digestive system and promoting stable blood sugar levels.

By following these nutritional guidelines and incorporating the recommended supplements, you can improve your health, achieve hormonal balance, and effectively manage your weight while following the Galveston Diet.

Chapter 2

30-Day Galveston Diet Meal Plan

Days 1-10

Day	Breakfast	Lunch	Dinner	Snack
1	Spinach and Feta Omelet (Page 10)	Grilled Chicken and Avocado Salad (Page 31)	Baked Salmon with Quinoa and Asparagus (Page 52)	Almond and Coconut Energy Balls (Page 70)
2	Greek Yogurt with Mixed Berries and Chia Seeds (Page 11)	Tuna Salad with Olive Oil and Lemon (Page 32)	Stuffed Bell Peppers with Ground Turkey and Black Beans (Page 53)	Celery Sticks with Almond Butter (Page 71)
3	Smoked Salmon and Avocado Scramble (Page 12)	Turkey and Spinach Lettuce Wraps (Page 33)	Zucchini Lasagna with Ground Beef (Page 54)	Cheese and Turkey Roll-Ups (Page 72)
4	Protein-Packed Smoothie with Almond Milk and Kale (Page 13)	Quinoa and Black Bean Salad with Lime Dressing (Page 34)	Baked Cod with Spinach and Brown Rice (Page 55)	Cucumber Slices with Hummus (Page 73)
5	Turkey Sausage and Egg Muffins (Page 14)	Shrimp and Avocado Stuffed Bell Peppers (Page 35)	Chickpea and Vegetable Curry (Page 56)	Greek Yogurt with Blueberries (Page 74)
6	Cottage Cheese with Pineapple and Walnuts (Page 15)	Smoked Salmon and Cucumber Roll-Ups (Page 36)	Grilled Shrimp with Cauliflower Rice Pilaf (Page 57)	Mixed Nuts and Seeds (Page 75)
7	Almond Butter Banana Protein Pancakes (Page 16)	Kale and Chicken Caesar Salad (Page 37)	Tofu and Vegetable Stir-Fry with Brown Rice (Page 58)	Hard-Boiled Eggs with Avocado (Page 76)
8	Chia Seed Pudding with Raspberries (Page 17)	Tofu and Veggie Stir-Fry with Sesame Oil (Page 38)	Baked Chicken with Broccoli and Quinoa (Page 59)	Bell Pepper Strips with Guacamole (Page 77)
9	Quinoa Breakfast Bowl with Blueberries and Almonds (Page 18)	Almond-Crusted Chicken Tenders (Page 39)	Stuffed Eggplant with Ground Lamb and Lentils (Page 60)	Turkey and Cheese Lettuce Wraps (Page 78)
10	Spinach and Mushroom Frittata (Page 19)	Spinach and Goat Cheese Stuffed Chicken Breast (Page 40)	Roasted Vegetable and Chickpea Bowl (Page 61)	Almond Flour Crackers with Cheese (Page 79)

Days 11-20

Day	Breakfast	Lunch	Dinner	Snack
11	Turkey Bacon and Avocado Egg Wrap (Page 20)	Salmon and Avocado Salad with Balsamic Vinaigrette (Page 41)	Grilled Pork Chops with Apple and Brussels Sprout Slaw (Page 62)	Cherry Tomatoes with Mozzarella Balls (Page 80)
12	Coconut Flour Pancakes with Strawberries (Page 21)	Egg Salad Lettuce Wraps (Page 42)	Baked Haddock with Spinach and Quinoa (Page 63)	Sliced Apple with Almond Butter (Page 81)
13	Veggie-Stuffed Bell Pepper with Eggs (Page 22)	Grilled Tuna and Mango Salsa (Page 43)	Black Bean and Sweet Potato Enchiladas (Page 64)	Greek Yogurt and Cucumber Dip (Page 82)
14	Greek Yogurt and Flaxseed Smoothie (Page 23)	Chicken and Asparagus Stir-Fry with Coconut Aminos (Page 44)	Grilled Steak with Asparagus and Wild Rice (Page 65)	Zucchini Chips with Greek Yogurt Dip (Page 83)
15	Egg White and Spinach Breakfast Burrito (Page 24)	Beef and Avocado Salad with Lime Cilantro Dressing (Page 45)	Veggie and Quinoa Stuffed Bell Peppers (Page 66)	Avocado and Cucumber Sushi Rolls (Page 84)
16	Avocado and Poached Egg on Whole Grain Toast (Page 25)	Zucchini Noodles with Pesto and Grilled Chicken (Page 46)	Chicken and Vegetable Skewers with Brown Rice (Page 67)	Smoked Salmon and Cream Cheese Cucumber Bites (Page 85)
17	Protein-Packed Overnight Oats with Chia Seeds (Page 26)	Turkey and Avocado Stuffed Tomatoes (Page 47)	Eggplant and Lentil Moussaka (Page 68)	Roasted Chickpeas with Spices (Page 86)
18	Broccoli and Cheddar Egg Cups (Page 27)	Quinoa and Kale Salad with Feta Cheese (Page 48)	Baked Salmon with Quinoa and Asparagus (Page 52)	Baked Kale Chips (Page 87)
19	Almond Milk and Berry Smoothie Bowl (Page 28)	Grilled Chicken and Broccoli Bowl with Tahini Dressing (Page 49)	Stuffed Bell Peppers with Ground Turkey and Black Beans (Page 53)	Radish and Carrot Sticks with Tzatziki (Page 88)
20	Chicken and Veggie Breakfast Skillet (Page 29)	Shrimp and Spinach Salad with Lemon Garlic Dressing (Page 50)	Zucchini Lasagna with Ground Beef (Page 54)	Sliced Bell Peppers with Tuna Salad (Page 89)

Days 21-30

Day	Breakfast	Lunch	Dinner	Snack
21	Spinach and Feta Omelet (Page 10)	Grilled Chicken and Avocado Salad (Page 31)	Baked Cod with Spinach and Brown Rice (Page 55)	Almond and Coconut Energy Balls (Page 70)
22	Greek Yogurt with Mixed Berries and Chia Seeds (Page 11)	Tuna Salad with Olive Oil and Lemon (Page 32)	Chickpea and Vegetable Curry (Page 56)	Celery Sticks with Almond Butter (Page 71)
23	Smoked Salmon and Avocado Scramble (Page 12)	Turkey and Spinach Lettuce Wraps (Page 33)	Grilled Shrimp with Cauliflower Rice Pilaf (Page 57)	Cheese and Turkey Roll-Ups (Page 72)
24	Protein-Packed Smoothie with Almond Milk and Kale (Page 13)	Quinoa and Black Bean Salad with Lime Dressing (Page 34)	Tofu and Vegetable Stir-Fry with Brown Rice (Page 58)	Cucumber Slices with Hummus (Page 73)
25	Turkey Sausage and Egg Muffins (Page 14)	Shrimp and Avocado Stuffed Bell Peppers (Page 35)	Baked Chicken with Broccoli and Quinoa (Page 59)	Greek Yogurt with Blueberries (Page 74)
26	Cottage Cheese with Pineapple and Walnuts (Page 15)	Smoked Salmon and Cucumber Roll-Ups (Page 36)	Stuffed Eggplant with Ground Lamb and Lentils (Page 60)	Mixed Nuts and Seeds (Page 75)
27	Almond Butter Banana Protein Pancakes (Page 16)	Kale and Chicken Caesar Salad (Page 37)	Roasted Vegetable and Chickpea Bowl (Page 61)	Hard-Boiled Eggs with Avocado (Page 76)
28	Chia Seed Pudding with Raspberries (Page 17)	Tofu and Veggie Stir-Fry with Sesame Oil (Page 38)	Grilled Pork Chops with Apple and Brussels Sprout Slaw (Page 62)	Bell Pepper Strips with Guacamole (Page 77)
29	Quinoa Breakfast Bowl with Blueberries and Almonds (Page 18)	Almond-Crusted Chicken Tenders (Page 39)	Baked Haddock with Spinach and Quinoa (Page 63)	Turkey and Cheese Lettuce Wraps (Page 78)
30	Spinach and Mushroom Frittata (Page 19)	Spinach and Goat Cheese Stuffed Chicken Breast (Page 40)	Black Bean and Sweet Potato Enchiladas (Page 64)	Almond Flour Crackers with Cheese (Page

Chapter 3: High-Protein Breakfasts

Spinach and Feta Omelet

Prep Time: 10 minutes | **Cook Time:** 10 minutes | **Servings:** 2

Ingredients:

- 4 large eggs
- 1 cup fresh spinach leaves, chopped
- 1/4 cup crumbled feta cheese
- 1/4 cup diced tomatoes
- 1/4 cup diced red bell pepper
- 1/4 teaspoon dried oregano
- Salt and freshly ground black pepper, to taste
- 1 tablespoon olive oil

Instructions:

1. Chop the fresh spinach leaves.
2. Dice the tomatoes and red bell pepper.
3. In a bowl, whisk together the eggs, chopped spinach, crumbled feta cheese, diced tomatoes, diced red bell pepper, dried oregano, salt, and black pepper.
4. Heat olive oil in a non-stick skillet over medium heat.
5. Pour the egg mixture into the skillet, spreading it evenly.
6. Cook for 3-4 minutes or until the edges begin to set.
7. Carefully fold the omelet in half using a spatula.
8. Cook for another 2-3 minutes or until the omelet is cooked through and the cheese is melted.
9. Slide the omelet onto a serving plate.
10. Garnish with additional chopped herbs if desired.

Nutritional Information:

- **Calories:** 276 kcal
- **Fat:** 20g
- **Carbohydrates:** 6g
- **Protein:** 18g

<u>Greek Yogurt with Mixed Berries and Chia Seeds</u>

Prep Time: 5 minutes | **Cook Time:** 0 minutes | **Servings:** 2

Ingredients:

- 1 cup Greek yogurt
- 1/2 cup mixed berries (such as strawberries, blueberries, raspberries)
- 1 tablespoon chia seeds
- 1 tablespoon honey (optional)
- Fresh mint leaves for garnish (optional)

Instructions:

1. If using whole berries, rinse them under cold water and pat dry with a paper towel.
2. Divide the Greek yogurt evenly between two serving bowls.
3. Top each bowl with mixed berries and sprinkle chia seeds over the berries.
4. If desired, drizzle honey over the yogurt and berries.
5. Garnish with fresh mint leaves if using.

Nutritional Information:

- **Calories:** 180 kcal
- **Fat:** 6g
- **Carbohydrates:** 18g
- **Protein:** 15g

Smoked Salmon and Avocado Scramble

Prep Time: 10 minutes | **Cook Time:** 5 minutes | **Servings:** 2

Ingredients:

- 4 large eggs
- 2 oz smoked salmon, chopped
- 1/2 avocado, diced
- 1 tablespoon chopped fresh dill
- Salt and freshly ground black pepper, to taste
- 1 tablespoon olive oil

Instructions:

1. Chop the smoked salmon into small pieces.
2. Dice the avocado into small cubes.
3. Chop the fresh dill.
4. In a bowl, whisk together the eggs, chopped smoked salmon, diced avocado, chopped fresh dill, salt, and black pepper.
5. Heat olive oil in a non-stick skillet over medium heat.
6. Pour the egg mixture into the skillet.
7. Cook, stirring gently with a spatula, until the eggs are scrambled and cooked to your desired consistency, about 3-4 minutes.
8. Divide the scrambled eggs onto plates.
9. Garnish with additional fresh dill if desired.

Nutritional Information:

- **Calories:** 315 kcal
- **Fat:** 24g
- **Carbohydrates:** 5g
- **Protein:** 21g

Protein-Packed Smoothie with Almond Milk and Kale

Prep Time: 5 minutes | **Cook Time:** 0 minutes | **Servings:** 2

Ingredients:

- 1 cup unsweetened almond milk

- 1/2 cup plain Greek yogurt

- 1 cup chopped kale leaves, stems removed

- 1/2 cup frozen berries (such as strawberries, blueberries)

- 1 tablespoon chia seeds

- 1 tablespoon almond butter

- 1 teaspoon honey (optional)

Instructions:

1. Chop the kale leaves, removing the stems.

2. In a blender, combine the unsweetened almond milk, plain Greek yogurt, chopped kale leaves, frozen berries, chia seeds, almond butter, and honey if using.

3. Blend until smooth and well combined, scraping down the sides of the blender as needed.

4. Pour the smoothie into glasses and serve immediately.

Nutritional Information:

- **Calories:** 220 kcal

- **Fat:** 11g

- **Carbohydrates:** 18g

- **Protein:** 15g

Turkey Sausage and Egg Muffins

Prep Time: 10 minutes | **Cook Time:** 20 minutes | **Servings:** 6 muffins

Ingredients:

- 6 large eggs
- 1/2-poundlean turkey sausage, casings removed
- 1/2 cup chopped bell peppers (any color)
- 1/4 cup chopped onion
- 1/4 cup chopped spinach
- Salt and freshly ground black pepper, to taste
- Cooking spray or olive oil for greasing

Instructions:

1. Preheat the oven to 350°F (175°C).

2. Take out the casings from the turkey sausage if needed.

3. Chop the bell peppers, onion, and spinach.

4. Heat a non-stick skillet over medium-high heat and lightly coat with cooking spray or olive oil.

5. Add the turkey sausage to the skillet, breaking it into small pieces with a spatula. Cook until browned and cooked through, about 5-7 minutes.

6. Add the chopped bell peppers and onion to the skillet with the sausage. Cook for another 2-3 minutes until the vegetables are softened.

7. Stir in the chopped spinach and cook until wilted, about 1 minute. Season with salt and pepper to taste. Remove from heat and let cool slightly.

8. In a mixing bowl, crack the eggs and whisk until well combined.

9. Add the cooked turkey sausage and vegetable mixture to the eggs, stirring to combine evenly.

10. Grease a muffin tin with cooking spray or olive oil.

11. Divide the egg mixture evenly among the muffin cups.

12. Bake in the preheated oven for 15-20 minutes, or until the muffins are set and lightly golden on top.

13. Remove from the oven and let cool slightly before serving.

14. Store leftovers in an airtight container in the refrigerator for up to 4 days.

Nutritional Information:

- **Calories:** 160 kcal
- **Fat:** 9g
- **Carbohydrates:** 3g
- **Protein:** 15g

Cottage Cheese with Pineapple and Walnuts

Prep Time: 5 minutes | **Cook Time:** 0 minutes | **Servings:** 2

Ingredients:

- 1 cup low-fat cottage cheese
- 1 cup fresh pineapple chunks
- 1/4 cup chopped walnuts

Instructions:

1. Chop the fresh pineapple into bite-sized chunks.
2. Chop the walnuts.
3. Divide the low-fat cottage cheese evenly between two serving bowls or plates.
4. Top each portion of cottage cheese with half of the fresh pineapple chunks.
5. Sprinkle each serving with half of the chopped walnuts.
6. Serve immediately as a nutritious snack or light meal.

Nutritional Information:

- **Calories:** 250 kcal
- **Fat:** 10g
- **Carbohydrates:** 22g
- **Protein:** 20g

Almond Butter Banana Protein Pancakes

Prep Time: 10 minutes | **Cook Time:** 10 minutes | **Servings:** 2

Ingredients:

- 1 large ripe banana
- 2 large eggs
- 2 tablespoons almond butter
- 1/2 teaspoon vanilla extract
- 1/2 teaspoon ground cinnamon
- 1/4 teaspoon baking powder
- Pinch of salt
- Olive oil or coconut oil, for cooking

Instructions:

1. In a mixing bowl, mash the ripe banana until smooth.

2. Add the eggs, almond butter, vanilla extract, ground cinnamon, baking powder, and a pinch of salt to the bowl.

3. Whisk all the ingredients together until well combined and smooth.

4. Heat a non-stick skillet or griddle over medium heat. Lightly grease the skillet with olive oil or coconut oil.

5. Pour about 1/4 cup of batter onto the skillet for each pancake. Cook until bubbles form on the surface of the pancake and the edges look set, about 2-3 minutes.

6. Carefully flip the pancakes and cook on the other side until golden brown and cooked through, about 1-2 minutes more.

7. Serve the pancakes warm, topped with fresh berries or a drizzle of almond butter if desired.

Nutritional Information:

- **Calories:** 330 kcal
- **Fat:** 21g
- **Carbohydrates:** 26g
- **Protein:** 14g

Chia Seed Pudding with Raspberries

Prep Time: 5 minutes | **Cook Time:** 0 minutes | **Servings:** 2

Ingredients:

- 1/4 cup chia seeds
- 1 cup unsweetened almond milk
- 1/2 teaspoon vanilla extract
- 1 tablespoon honey or maple syrup (optional, adjust to taste)
- 1 cup fresh raspberries
- 2 tablespoons chopped walnuts (optional)

Instructions:

1. In a mixing bowl or jar, combine chia seeds, unsweetened almond milk, vanilla extract, and honey or maple syrup (if using). Stir adequately to combine.

2. Cover the bowl or jar and refrigerate for at least 2 hours, or preferably overnight, to allow the chia seeds to absorb the liquid and thicken into a pudding-like consistency.

3. Once the chia pudding has thickened, divide it into serving bowls or glasses.

4. Top each serving with fresh raspberries and chopped walnuts, if desired.

Nutritional Information:

- **Calories:** 240 kcal
- **Fat:** 11g
- **Carbohydrates:** 30g
- **Protein:** 7g

Quinoa Breakfast Bowl with Blueberries and Almonds

Prep Time: 5 minutes | **Cook Time:** 15 minutes | **Servings:** 2

Ingredients:

- 1/2 cup quinoa
- 1 cup water or unsweetened almond milk
- 1/2 teaspoon vanilla extract
- 1/2 teaspoon ground cinnamon
- 1 tablespoon honey or maple syrup (optional, adjust to taste)
- 1/2 cup fresh blueberries
- 2 tablespoons sliced almonds
- Fresh mint leaves for garnish (optional)

Instructions:

1. Rinse the quinoa under cold water until the water runs clear.
2. In a saucepan, bring the water or almond milk to a boil. Add the rinsed quinoa, reduce heat to low, cover, and simmer for about 15 minutes, or until all the liquid is absorbed and the quinoa is fluffy.
3. Once cooked, stir in the vanilla extract, ground cinnamon, and honey or maple syrup (if using), ensuring it is evenly mixed.
4. Divide the cooked quinoa into serving bowls.
5. Top each bowl with fresh blueberries and sliced almonds.
6. Garnish with fresh mint leaves if desired.
7. Enjoy warm.

Nutritional Information:

- **Calories:** 280 kcal
- **Fat:** 9g
- **Carbohydrates:** 45g
- **Protein:** 8g

Spinach and Mushroom Frittata

Prep Time: 10 minutes | **Cook Time:** 20 minutes | **Servings:** 4

Ingredients:

- 8 large eggs
- 1/4 cup unsweetened almond milk
- 1 cup fresh spinach, chopped
- 1 cup mushrooms, sliced
- 1/2 cup cherry tomatoes, halved
- 1/4 cup onions, finely chopped
- 1 clove garlic, minced
- 1/4 cup feta cheese, crumbled
- 1 tablespoon olive oil
- 1/2 teaspoon salt
- 1/4 teaspoon black pepper

Instructions:

1. Preheat your oven to 375 degrees Fahrenheit (190 degrees Celsius).
2. In a large oven-safe skillet, heat the olive oil over medium heat.
3. Add the finely chopped onions and minced garlic, sautéing until fragrant and translucent, about 2-3 minutes.
4. Add the sliced mushrooms and continue to sauté until they release their moisture and begin to brown, about 5 minutes.
5. Stir in the chopped spinach and cook until wilted, about 2 minutes.
6. Add the halved cherry tomatoes and cook for another minute. Take out the skillet from heat.
7. In a large bowl, whisk together the eggs, unsweetened almond milk, salt, and black pepper.
8. Pour the egg mixture over the cooked vegetables in the skillet.
9. Sprinkle the crumbled feta cheese evenly over the top.
10. Transfer the skillet to the preheated oven.
11. Bake for 15-20 minutes, or until the eggs are set and the top is lightly browned.
12. Remove from the oven and let it cool for a few minutes before slicing and serving.

Nutritional Information (per serving):

- **Calories:** 210 kcal
- **Fat:** 14g
- **Carbohydrates:** 5g
- **Protein:** 16g

Turkey Bacon and Avocado Egg Wrap

Prep Time: 10 minutes | **Cook Time:** 10 minutes | **Servings:** 2

Ingredients:

- 4 large eggs
- 4 slices turkey bacon
- 1 avocado, sliced
- 1 cup spinach, fresh
- 2 whole grain tortillas
- 1/4 cup feta cheese, crumbled
- 1 tablespoon olive oil
- 1/4 teaspoon salt
- 1/4 teaspoon black pepper

Instructions:

1. In a skillet over medium heat, cook the turkey bacon slices until crispy, about 5-7 minutes. Remove from the skillet and set aside on a paper towel-lined plate.

2. In the same skillet, heat the olive oil over medium heat.

3. Crack the eggs into the skillet and scramble them, adding salt and black pepper to taste. Cook until the eggs are just set, about 3-4 minutes.

4. Warm the whole grain tortillas in a dry skillet or microwave.

5. Place half of the fresh spinach in the center of each tortilla.

6. Divide the scrambled eggs evenly between the tortillas, placing them on top of the spinach.

7. Add two slices of cooked turkey bacon to each wrap.

8. Top with the sliced avocado and crumbled feta cheese.

9. Fold in the sides of the tortillas and roll them up to form wraps.

10. Cut each wrap in half and serve immediately.

Nutritional Information (per serving):

- **Calories:** 350 kcal
- **Fat:** 20g
- **Carbohydrates:** 20g
- **Protein:** 24g

Coconut Flour Pancakes with Strawberries

Prep Time: 10 minutes | **Cook Time:** 10 minutes | **Servings:** 2

Ingredients:

- 1/4 cup coconut flour
- 1/2 teaspoon baking powder
- 1/4 teaspoon salt
- 4 large eggs
- 1/4 cup unsweetened almond milk
- 1 tablespoon coconut oil, melted
- 1 teaspoon vanilla extract
- 1 cup strawberries, sliced
- 1 tablespoon coconut oil (for cooking)

Instructions:

1. In a mixing bowl, combine the coconut flour, baking powder, and salt.
2. In a separate bowl, whisk the eggs, unsweetened almond milk, melted coconut oil, and vanilla extract.
3. Gradually add the wet ingredients to the dry ingredients, mixing until a smooth batter forms.
4. Heat a non-stick skillet over medium heat and add 1 tablespoon of coconut oil.
5. Pour 1/4 cup of the batter onto the skillet for each pancake.
6. Cook until bubbles form on the surface and the edges begin to set, about 2-3 minutes.
7. Flip the pancakes and cook for another 2-3 minutes until golden brown and cooked through.
8. Plate the pancakes and top with the sliced strawberries.

Nutritional Information (per serving):

- **Calories:** 320 kcal
- **Fat:** 22g
- **Carbohydrates:** 15g
- **Protein:** 14g

Veggie-Stuffed Bell Pepper with Eggs

Prep Time: 15 minutes | **Cook Time:** 25 minutes | **Servings:** 4

Ingredients:

- 4 large bell peppers, tops cut off and seeds removed
- 1 tablespoon olive oil
- 1 small onion, diced
- 1 cup mushrooms, sliced
- 1 cup spinach, chopped
- 1 small zucchini, diced
- 1/2 cup cherry tomatoes, halved
- 6 large eggs
- 1/4 cup unsweetened almond milk
- 1/4 teaspoon salt
- 1/4 teaspoon black pepper
- 1/4 cup feta cheese, crumbled (optional)
- Fresh basil, chopped (for garnish)

Instructions:

1. Preheat the oven to 375°F (190°C).
2. Place the bell peppers, cut side up, in a baking dish.
3. Heat the olive oil in a large skillet over medium heat.
4. Add the diced onion and cook until softened, about 3 minutes.
5. Add the sliced mushrooms and cook for another 5 minutes until they start to brown.
6. Add the chopped spinach, diced zucchini, and halved cherry tomatoes. Cook for another 3 minutes until the vegetables are tender.
7. In a mixing bowl, whisk together the eggs, unsweetened almond milk, salt, and black pepper.
8. Evenly distribute the cooked vegetables into the prepared bell peppers.
9. Pour the egg mixture over the vegetables in each bell pepper.
10. Sprinkle crumbled feta cheese on top if using.
11. Place the baking dish in the preheated oven and bake for 25 minutes, or until the eggs are set and the bell peppers are tender.
12. Garnish with fresh chopped basil before serving.

Nutritional Information (per serving):

- **Calories:** 210 kcal
- **Fat:** 14g
- **Carbohydrates:** 8g
- **Protein:** 12g

Greek Yogurt and Flaxseed Smoothie

Prep Time: 5 minutes | **Cook Time:** 0 minutes | **Servings:** 2

Ingredients:

- 1 cup Greek yogurt
- 1 cup unsweetened almond milk
- 1 medium banana, sliced
- 1 cup fresh or frozen berries (e.g., blueberries, strawberries)
- 1 tablespoon ground flaxseed
- 1 tablespoon chia seeds
- 1 teaspoon vanilla extract
- 1 handful spinach leaves, washed
- 1 tablespoon almond butter

Instructions:

1. Slice the banana.
2. Wash the spinach leaves.
3. In a blender, combine the Greek yogurt, unsweetened almond milk, sliced banana, fresh or frozen berries, ground flaxseed, chia seeds, vanilla extract, spinach leaves, and almond butter.
4. Blend until smooth and creamy.
5. Pour the smoothie into two glasses and serve immediately.

Nutritional Information (per serving):

- **Calories:** 210 kcal
- **Fat:** 11g
- **Carbohydrates:** 18g
- **Protein:** 12g

Egg White and Spinach Breakfast Burrito

Prep Time: 10 minutes | **Cook Time:** 10 minutes | **Servings:** 2

Ingredients:

- 1 cup egg whites
- 1 cup fresh spinach leaves, washed and chopped
- 1/2 cup bell pepper, diced
- 1/4 cup red onion, finely chopped
- 1 tablespoon olive oil
- 2 whole wheat tortillas
- 1/4 cup shredded low-fat cheese
- 1 small avocado, sliced
- Salt and pepper to taste

Instructions:

1. Wash and chop the spinach leaves.
2. Dice the bell pepper.
3. Finely chop the red onion.
4. Slice the avocado.
5. Heat the olive oil in a non-stick skillet over medium heat.
6. Add the diced bell pepper and finely chopped red onion to the skillet and sauté until softened, about 3-4 minutes.
7. Add the chopped spinach leaves and cook until wilted, about 1-2 minutes.
8. Pour the egg whites into the skillet with the vegetables.
9. Cook, stirring frequently, until the egg whites are fully cooked and no longer runny, about 3-4 minutes.
10. Season with salt and pepper to taste.
11. Warm the whole wheat tortillas in a separate skillet or microwave.
12. Divide the egg white and vegetable mixture evenly between the two tortillas.
13. Sprinkle the shredded low-fat cheese over the egg mixture.
14. Add the sliced avocado on top.
15. Roll up each tortilla to form a burrito.
16. Serve the breakfast burritos immediately.

Nutritional Information (per serving):

- **Calories:** 275 kcal
- **Fat:** 12g
- **Carbohydrates:** 24g
- **Protein:** 18g

Avocado and Poached Egg on Whole Grain Toast

Prep Time: 10 minutes | **Cook Time:** 5 minutes | **Servings:** 2

Ingredients:

- 2 large eggs
- 1 ripe avocado, mashed
- 2 slices whole grain bread
- 1 tablespoon lemon juice
- Salt and pepper to taste
- 1 tablespoon olive oil
- Optional: red pepper flakes for garnish

Instructions:

1. Mash the ripe avocado in a bowl.
2. Add lemon juice, salt, and pepper to the mashed avocado and mix adequately.
3. Toast the whole grain bread slices until golden brown.
4. Bring a pot of water to a gentle simmer.
5. Add a splash of vinegar to the water (optional).
6. Crack each egg into a small bowl.
7. Carefully slide the eggs into the simmering water.
8. Poach the eggs for about 3-4 minutes, until the whites are set but the yolks are still runny.
9. Use a slotted spoon to take out the poached eggs from the water and place them on a paper towel to drain.
10. Spread the mashed avocado mixture evenly on each slice of toasted whole grain bread.
11. Place a poached egg on top of each slice of avocado toast.
12. Drizzle olive oil over the top.
13. Garnish with red pepper flakes, if using.
14. Season with additional salt and pepper to taste.

Nutritional Information (per serving):

- **Calories:** 275 kcal
- **Fat:** 19g
- **Carbohydrates:** 20g
- **Protein:** 10g

Protein-Packed Overnight Oats with Chia Seeds

Prep Time: 10 minutes | **Cook Time:** 0 minutes (overnight soak) | **Servings:** 2

Ingredients:

- 1 cup rolled oats
- 1 cup unsweetened almond milk
- 1/2 cup Greek yogurt, plain
- 2 tablespoons chia seeds
- 1 tablespoon flaxseeds, ground
- 1 tablespoon honey
- 1/2 teaspoon vanilla extract
- 1/2 cup mixed berries, fresh or frozen
- 1/4 cup chopped nuts (almonds, walnuts, or pecans)

Instructions:

1. In a medium-sized bowl, combine rolled oats, unsweetened almond milk, plain Greek yogurt, chia seeds, ground flaxseeds, honey, and vanilla extract. Stir adequately to ensure all ingredients are evenly mixed.

2. Gently fold in the fresh or frozen mixed berries.

3. Cover the bowl with a lid or plastic wrap and refrigerate overnight (or for at least 4 hours) to allow the oats and chia seeds to absorb the liquid and soften.

4. In the morning, give the oats a good stir. If the mixture is too thick, add a splash of unsweetened almond milk to reach your desired consistency.

5. Divide the overnight oats into two servings. Top each serving with chopped nuts.

Nutritional Information (per serving):

- **Calories:** 290 kcal
- **Fat:** 12g
- **Carbohydrates:** 35g
- **Protein:** 12g

Broccoli and Cheddar Egg Cups

Prep Time: 15 minutes | **Cook Time:** 20 minutes | **Servings:** 6

Ingredients:

- 6 large eggs
- 1 cup broccoli florets, finely chopped
- 1/2 cup cheddar cheese, shredded
- 1/4 cup onion, finely diced
- 1/4 cup red bell pepper, finely diced
- 1/4 cup almond milk, unsweetened
- 1/2 teaspoon salt
- 1/4 teaspoon black pepper
- 1 tablespoon olive oil

Instructions:

1. Preheat your oven to 350 degrees Fahrenheit (175 degrees Celsius).
2. Grease a 12-cup muffin tin with olive oil.
3. In a skillet over medium heat, add olive oil and sauté the finely diced onion and red bell pepper until they are soft, about 3-4 minutes.
4. Add the finely chopped broccoli florets and cook for an additional 2-3 minutes until tender. Set aside to cool slightly.
5. In a large bowl, whisk together the large eggs, unsweetened almond milk, salt, and black pepper.
6. Add the sautéed vegetables and shredded cheddar cheese to the egg mixture. Stir until well combined.
7. Divide the mixture evenly among the 12 muffin cups, filling each about three-quarters full.
8. Bake in the preheated oven for 18-20 minutes, or until the egg cups are set and lightly golden on top.
9. Allow the egg cups to cool in the muffin tin for a few minutes before removing. Serve warm.

Nutritional Information (per serving):

- **Calories:** 150 kcal
- **Fat:** 10g
- **Carbohydrates:** 5g
- **Protein:** 10g

Almond Milk and Berry Smoothie Bowl

Prep Time: 10 minutes | **Cook Time:** 0 minutes | **Servings:** 2

Ingredients:

- 1 cup unsweetened almond milk
- 1 cup mixed berries, frozen
- 1 medium banana, sliced and frozen
- 1 tablespoon chia seeds
- 1 tablespoon almond butter
- 1/2 teaspoon vanilla extract
- 1/4 cup Greek yogurt, plain
- 1/4 cup granola, low sugar
- 2 tablespoons sliced almonds
- 1/4 cup fresh berries (for topping)
- 2 tablespoons shredded coconut, unsweetened

Instructions:

1. In a blender, combine the unsweetened almond milk, frozen mixed berries, sliced frozen banana, chia seeds, almond butter, vanilla extract, and plain Greek yogurt. Blend until smooth and creamy.

2. Pour the smoothie mixture into two bowls.

3. Top each bowl with low-sugar granola, sliced almonds, fresh berries, and shredded coconut.

Nutritional Information (per serving):

- **Calories:** 250 kcal
- **Fat:** 12g
- **Carbohydrates:** 30g
- **Protein:** 10g

Chicken and Veggie Breakfast Skillet

Prep Time: 15 minutes | **Cook Time:** 20 minutes | **Servings:** 4

Ingredients:

- 1 tablespoon olive oil
- 1 pound boneless, skinless chicken breasts, cut into bite-sized pieces
- 1 medium onion, chopped
- 1 red bell pepper, chopped
- 1 green bell pepper, chopped
- 2 cloves garlic, minced
- 1 teaspoon paprika
- 1/2 teaspoon dried thyme
- 1/2 teaspoon dried oregano
- Salt and pepper, to taste
- 2 cups spinach leaves
- 1 cup cherry tomatoes, halved
- 4 large eggs
- Fresh parsley, chopped (for garnish)

Instructions:

1. Heat olive oil in a large skillet over medium-high heat. Add chicken pieces and cook until browned and cooked through, about 5-7 minutes. Remove chicken from skillet and set aside.

2. In the same skillet, add chopped onion, red bell pepper, and green bell pepper. Cook until vegetables are softened, about 5 minutes.

3. Add minced garlic, paprika, dried thyme, dried oregano, salt, and pepper. Stir and cook for another minute until fragrant.

4. Reduce heat to medium. Add spinach leaves and cherry tomatoes to the skillet. Stir until spinach is wilted and tomatoes are heated through, about 2-3 minutes.

5. Create 4 wells in the vegetable mixture using a spoon. Crack one egg into each well.

6. Cover the skillet with a lid and cook until eggs are cooked to desired doneness, about 5-7 minutes for runny yolks or longer for fully cooked yolks.

7. Sprinkle with chopped fresh parsley before serving.

Nutritional Information (per serving):

- **Calories:** 280 kcal
- **Fat:** 12g
- **Carbohydrates:** 9g
- **Protein:** 32g

Chapter 4: Healthy Fats & Protein Lunches

Grilled Chicken and Avocado Salad

Prep Time: 15 minutes | **Cook Time:** 15 minutes | **Total Time:** 30 minutes | **Servings:** 4

Ingredients:

- 1-poundboneless, skinless chicken breasts
- 2 avocados, diced
- 4 cups mixed salad greens
- 1 cup cherry tomatoes, halved
- 1/2 red onion, thinly sliced
- 1/4 cup chopped fresh cilantro
- Juice of 1 lime
- 2 tablespoons olive oil
- Salt and pepper to taste

Instructions:

1. Preheat grill to medium-high heat. Season chicken breasts with salt and pepper. Grill for about 6-7 minutes per side, or until cooked through (internal temperature of 165°F). Let rest for 5 minutes before slicing into strips.

2. In a large bowl, combine the mixed salad greens, cherry tomatoes, red onion, diced avocado, and cilantro.

3. In a small bowl, whisk together lime juice, olive oil, salt, and pepper.

4. Add the grilled chicken strips to the salad. Drizzle with the dressing and toss gently to combine.

Nutritional Information:

- **Calories:** 320 kcal
- **Fat:** 18g
- **Carbohydrates:** 12g
- **Protein:** 28g

Tuna Salad with Olive Oil and Lemon

Prep Time: 10 minutes | **Cook Time:** 0 minutes | **Total Time:** 10 minutes | **Servings:** 2

Ingredients:

- 2 cans (5 oz each) tuna, drained
- 1/4 cup diced cucumber
- 1/4 cup diced red bell pepper
- 1/4 cup diced red onion
- 1/4 cup chopped fresh parsley
- Juice of 1 lemon
- 2 tablespoons extra virgin olive oil
- Salt and pepper to taste
- Mixed salad greens for serving

Instructions:

1. In a mixing bowl, combine the drained tuna, diced cucumber, diced red bell pepper, diced red onion, and chopped parsley.
2. In a small bowl, whisk together the lemon juice, extra virgin olive oil, salt, and pepper.
3. Pour the dressing over the tuna mixture and toss gently to coat.
4. Divide the mixed salad greens onto plates. Top with the tuna salad mixture.

Nutritional Information:

- **Calories:** 280 kcal
- **Fat:** 15g
- **Carbohydrates:** 6g
- **Protein:** 30g

Turkey and Spinach Lettuce Wraps

Prep Time: 15 minutes | **Cook Time:** 10 minutes | **Total Time:** 25 minutes | **Servings:** 4

Ingredients:

- 1-poundground turkey
- 1 tablespoon olive oil
- 2 cloves garlic, minced
- 1 teaspoon ground cumin
- 1 teaspoon paprika
- 1/2 teaspoon chili powder
- Salt and pepper to taste
- 2 cups fresh spinach leaves
- 1/2 cup diced red bell pepper
- 1/4 cup diced red onion
- 1/4 cup chopped fresh cilantro
- Juice of 1 lime
- 8 large lettuce leaves (such as butter lettuce or romaine)

Instructions:

1. In a large skillet, heat olive oil over medium heat. Add minced garlic and cook for 1 minute until fragrant. Add ground turkey, cumin, paprika, chili powder, salt, and pepper. Cook until turkey is browned and cooked through, about 7-8 minutes, breaking it up with a spoon as it cooks.

2. Add spinach leaves, diced red bell pepper, diced red onion, and chopped cilantro to the skillet with the cooked turkey. Stir and cook for 2-3 minutes until the spinach is wilted and the vegetables are tender. Remove from heat.

3. Squeeze the juice of 1 lime over the turkey and vegetable mixture. Stir to combine.

4. Spoon the turkey and vegetable mixture onto each lettuce leaf. Roll up the lettuce leaves to form wraps.

5. Arrange the lettuce wraps on a serving platter and serve immediately.

Nutritional Information:

- **Calories:** 250 kcal
- **Fat:** 12g
- **Carbohydrates:** 8g
- **Protein:** 28g

Quinoa and Black Bean Salad with Lime Dressing

Prep Time: 15 minutes | **Cook Time:** 15 minutes | **Total Time:** 30 minutes | **Servings:** 4

Ingredients:

- 1 cup quinoa, rinsed
- 1 can (15 oz) black beans, drained and rinsed
- 1 cup diced red bell pepper
- 1/2 cup diced red onion
- 1/4 cup chopped fresh cilantro
- Juice of 2 limes
- 3 tablespoons extra virgin olive oil
- 1 teaspoon ground cumin
- Salt and pepper to taste
- Mixed salad greens for serving

Instructions:

1. In a medium saucepan, combine quinoa with 2 cups of water. Bring to a boil, then reduce heat to low, cover, and simmer for 12-15 minutes, or until quinoa is cooked and water is absorbed. Remove from heat and let it cool.

2. In a large bowl, combine cooked quinoa, black beans, diced red bell pepper, diced red onion, and chopped cilantro.

3. In a small bowl, whisk together lime juice, extra virgin olive oil, ground cumin, salt, and pepper.

4. Pour the dressing over the quinoa and black bean mixture. Toss gently to coat everything evenly.

5. Arrange mixed salad greens on plates or in bowls. Spoon the quinoa and black bean salad over the greens.

Nutritional Information:

- **Calories:** 320 kcal
- **Fat:** 12g
- **Carbohydrates:** 45g
- **Protein:** 12g

Shrimp and Avocado Stuffed Bell Peppers

Prep Time: 20 minutes | **Cook Time:** 20 minutes | **Total Time:** 40 minutes | **Servings:** 4

Ingredients:

- 4 bell peppers (any color), tops cut off and seeds removed
- 1-poundshrimp, peeled and deveined
- 2 avocados, diced
- 1/2 cup diced cucumber
- 1/4 cup diced red onion
- 1/4 cup chopped fresh cilantro
- Juice of 1 lime
- 2 tablespoons extra virgin olive oil
- Salt and pepper to taste

Instructions:

1. Preheat oven to 375°F (190°C). Place the hollowed-out bell peppers on a baking sheet lined with parchment paper. Bake for 15-20 minutes until slightly softened.

2. In a large skillet, heat olive oil over medium-high heat. Add shrimp and cook for 3-4 minutes until pink and cooked through. Remove from heat and let cool slightly.

3. In a large bowl, combine diced avocado, diced cucumber, diced red onion, chopped cilantro, lime juice, salt, and pepper. Add the cooked shrimp and gently toss to combine.

4. Spoon the shrimp and avocado mixture into the precooked bell peppers, dividing evenly among them.

5. Arrange the stuffed bell peppers on a serving platter and serve immediately.

Nutritional Information:

- **Calories:** 320 kcal
- **Fat:** 18g
- **Carbohydrates:** 18g
- **Protein:** 25g

Smoked Salmon and Cucumber Roll-Ups

Prep Time: 15 minutes | **Cook Time:** 0 minutes | **Total Time:** 15 minutes | **Servings:** 4

Ingredients:

- 1 large cucumber
- 4 oz smoked salmon, thinly sliced
- 1/2 cup Greek yogurt or cream cheese
- 2 tablespoons chopped fresh dill
- Juice of 1/2 lemon
- Salt and pepper to taste

Instructions:

1. Using a vegetable peeler, slice the cucumber lengthwise into thin strips. Pat dry with paper towels to remove excess moisture.

2. In a small bowl, mix Greek yogurt or cream cheese with chopped fresh dill, lemon juice, salt, and pepper.

3. Lay out cucumber strips on a clean surface. Place a slice of smoked salmon on each cucumber strip. Spoon a small amount of the yogurt or cream cheese mixture onto each salmon slice.

4. Roll up each cucumber strip with the salmon and filling inside. Secure with a toothpick if necessary.

5. Arrange the smoked salmon and cucumber roll-ups on a serving platter.

Nutritional Information:

- **Calories:** 120 kcal
- **Fat:** 7g
- **Carbohydrates:** 4g
- **Protein:** 10g

Kale and Chicken Caesar Salad

Prep Time: 15 minutes | **Cook Time:** 15 minutes | **Total Time:** 30 minutes | **Servings:** 4

Ingredients:

- 1-poundboneless, skinless chicken breasts
- 1 bunch kale, stems removed and leaves chopped
- 1/2 cup cherry tomatoes, halved
- 1/4 cup grated Parmesan cheese
- 1/4 cup Caesar dressing (made with olive oil)
- Salt and pepper to taste

Instructions:

1. Season the chicken breasts with salt and pepper. Grill or pan-sear until cooked through, about 6-7 minutes per side. Let rest for 5 minutes before slicing thinly.

2. In a large bowl, massage the chopped kale with a little olive oil and a pinch of salt for a few minutes until the kale softens.

3. Add sliced chicken, cherry tomatoes, grated Parmesan cheese, and Caesar dressing to the bowl of kale.

4. Toss everything together until well combined and evenly coated with dressing.

5. Divide the salad among plates and serve immediately.

Nutritional Information:

- **Calories:** 320 kcal
- **Fat:** 18g
- **Carbohydrates:** 9g
- **Protein:** 30g

Tofu and Veggie Stir-Fry with Sesame Oil

Prep Time: 15 minutes | **Cook Time:** 15 minutes | **Total Time:** 30 minutes | **Servings:** 4

Ingredients:

- 14 oz block of firm tofu, drained and cut into cubes
- 1 red bell pepper, sliced
- 1 yellow bell pepper, sliced
- 1 cup broccoli florets
- 1 cup snap peas
- 2 cloves garlic, minced
- 1 tbsp grated fresh ginger
- 3 tbsp low-sodium soy sauce
-
- 1 tbsp sesame oil
- 1 tbsp rice vinegar
- 1 tbsp cornstarch
- 2 tbsp water
- Salt and pepper to taste
- Sesame seeds for garnish
- Cooked brown rice or quinoa, for serving

Instructions:

1. Press the tofu between paper towels or a clean kitchen towel to remove excess moisture. Cut into cubes and set aside.

2. Heat sesame oil in a large pan or wok over medium-high heat. Add minced garlic and grated ginger, stir-frying for about 30 seconds until fragrant.

3. Add tofu cubes to the pan and cook until lightly browned on all sides, about 5-7 minutes. Remove tofu from the pan and set aside.

4. In a small bowl, mix soy sauce, rice vinegar, cornstarch, and water until smooth.

5. In the same pan, stir-fry bell peppers, broccoli florets, and snap peas until crisp-tender, about 5 minutes.

6. Return tofu to the pan. Pour the sauce over the tofu and vegetables. Stir adequately to coat everything evenly. Cook for another 2-3 minutes until the sauce thickens.

7. Taste and season with salt and pepper if needed.

8. Serve the tofu and vegetable stir-fry over cooked brown rice or quinoa. Garnish with sesame seeds.

Nutritional Information:

- **Calories:** 280 kcal
- **Fat:** 12g
- **Carbohydrates:** 20g
- **Protein:** 25g

Almond-Crusted Chicken Tenders

Prep Time: 15 minutes | **Cook Time:** 20 minutes | **Total Time:** 35 minutes | **Servings:** 4

Ingredients:

- 1-poundchicken tenders
- 1 cup almond flour
- 1/2 cup finely chopped almonds
- 1/2 tsp garlic powder
- 1/2 tsp paprika
- 1/2 tsp salt
- 1/4 tsp black pepper
- 2 eggs, beaten
- Cooking spray or olive oil spray

Instructions:

1. Preheat the oven to 400°F (200°C). Line a baking sheet with parchment paper and lightly grease with cooking spray.

2. In a shallow bowl, combine almond flour, chopped almonds, garlic powder, paprika, salt, and black pepper. Mix adequately.

3. Dip each chicken tender first into the beaten eggs, then coat evenly with the almond mixture, pressing gently to adhere. Place the coated tenders on the prepared baking sheet.

4. Lightly spray the top of the chicken tenders with cooking spray or olive oil spray. Bake in the preheated oven for 15-20 minutes, or until the chicken is cooked through and the coating is golden brown and crispy.

5. Serve the almond-crusted chicken tenders warm with a side of mixed greens or steamed vegetables.

Nutritional Information:

- **Calories:** 350 kcal
- **Fat:** 21g
- **Carbohydrates:** 8g
- **Protein:** 32g

Spinach and Goat Cheese Stuffed Chicken Breast

Prep Time: 15 minutes | **Cook Time:** 25 minutes | **Total Time:** 40 minutes | **Servings:** 4

Ingredients:

- 4 boneless, skinless chicken breasts
- 2 cups fresh spinach leaves, chopped
- 1/2 cup crumbled goat cheese
- 2 cloves garlic, minced
- 1/2 tsp dried thyme
- Salt and pepper, to taste
- Olive oil cooking spray

Instructions:

1. Preheat the oven to 375°F (190°C). Lightly grease a baking dish with olive oil cooking spray.

2. Using a sharp knife, carefully cut a pocket into the side of each chicken breast without cutting all the way through.

3. In a mixing bowl, combine chopped spinach, crumbled goat cheese, minced garlic, dried thyme, salt, and pepper.

4. Spoon the spinach and goat cheese mixture evenly into the pockets of the chicken breasts, pressing gently to secure.

5. Place the stuffed chicken breasts in the prepared baking dish. Lightly spray the tops with olive oil cooking spray. Bake in the preheated oven for 20-25 minutes, or until the chicken is cooked through and reaches an internal temperature of 165°F (74°C).

6. Remove from the oven and let rest for a few minutes before serving. Optionally, garnish with additional fresh herbs if desired.

Nutritional Information:

- **Calories:** 280 kcal
- **Fat:** 12g
- **Carbohydrates:** 2g
- **Protein:** 40g

Salmon and Avocado Salad with Balsamic Vinaigrette

Prep Time: 15 minutes | **Cook Time:** 10 minutes | **Total Time:** 25 minutes | **Servings:** 4

Ingredients:

- 4 salmon fillets, skinless
- 1 avocado, sliced
- 4 cups mixed greens (spinach, arugula, lettuce)
- 1/2 cup cherry tomatoes, halved
- 1/4 cup red onion, thinly sliced
- 1/4 cup cucumber, thinly sliced
- 2 tbsp olive oil
- 2 tbsp balsamic vinegar
- 1 clove garlic, minced
- Salt and pepper, to taste

Instructions:

1. Preheat the oven to 400°F (200°C). Line a baking sheet with parchment paper.

2. Place the salmon fillets on the prepared baking sheet. Drizzle with 1 tablespoon of olive oil and season with salt and pepper. Bake for 10 minutes, or until the salmon is cooked through and flakes easily with a fork.

3. In a small bowl, whisk together the remaining olive oil, balsamic vinegar, minced garlic, salt, and pepper to make the vinaigrette.

4. In a large bowl, combine mixed greens, cherry tomatoes, red onion, and cucumber. Toss with half of the prepared vinaigrette.

5. Divide the salad mixture among serving plates. Top each plate with a baked salmon fillet and sliced avocado.

6. Drizzle the remaining vinaigrette over the salmon and avocado. Optionally, garnish with fresh herbs like parsley or dill if desired.

Nutritional Information:

- **Calories:** 320 kcal
- **Fat:** 20g
- **Carbohydrates:** 10g
- **Protein:** 25g

Egg Salad Lettuce Wraps

Prep Time: 15 minutes | **Cook Time:** 10 minutes | **Total Time:** 25 minutes | **Servings:** 4

Ingredients:

- 8 large eggs
- 1/4 cup Greek yogurt
- 1 tbsp Dijon mustard
- 1/4 cup celery, finely chopped
- 1/4 cup red bell pepper, finely chopped
- 2 tbsp red onion, finely chopped
- Salt and pepper, to taste
- 8 large lettuce leaves (such as Bibb or Romaine)

Instructions:

1. Place the eggs in a saucepan and cover with cold water. Bring to a boil over medium-high heat. Once boiling, cover, remove from heat, and let sit for 10 minutes. Drain and rinse under cold water. Peel the eggs and chop them finely.

2. In a mixing bowl, combine the chopped eggs, Greek yogurt, Dijon mustard, celery, red bell pepper, red onion, salt, and pepper. Mix adequately until everything is evenly combined.

3. Lay out the lettuce leaves on a clean surface. Spoon the egg salad mixture evenly among the lettuce leaves.

4. Carefully roll up each lettuce leaf, enclosing the filling like a burrito.

5. Arrange the lettuce wraps on a serving platter and serve immediately.

Nutritional Information:

- **Calories:** 190 kcal
- **Fat:** 12g
- **Carbohydrates:** 4g
- **Protein:** 15g

Grilled Tuna and Mango Salsa

Prep Time: 15 minutes | **Cook Time:** 10 minutes | **Total Time:** 25 minutes | **Servings:** 4

Ingredients:

- 4 tuna steaks (about 6 oz each)
- 2 mangoes, peeled and diced
- 1 red bell pepper, diced
- 1/4 cup red onion, finely chopped
- 1/4 cup fresh cilantro, chopped
- Juice of 1 lime
- 1 tbsp olive oil
- Salt and pepper, to taste

Instructions:

1. Preheat grill to medium-high heat.

2. Season tuna steaks with salt and pepper. Grill for about 4-5 minutes per side, or until desired doneness. Remove from grill and let rest.

3. In a bowl, combine diced mangoes, red bell pepper, red onion, cilantro, lime juice, olive oil, salt, and pepper. Mix adequately to combine.

4. Place grilled tuna steaks on plates and top generously with mango salsa.

5. Serve immediately, and enjoy your Grilled Tuna and Mango Salsa!

Nutritional Information:

- **Calories:** 320 kcal
- **Fat:** 12g
- **Carbohydrates:** 20g
- **Protein:** 32g

Chicken and Asparagus Stir-Fry with Coconut Aminos

Prep Time: 15 minutes | **Cook Time:** 15 minutes | **Total Time:** 30 minutes | **Servings:** 4

Ingredients:

- 1-poundboneless, skinless chicken breasts, thinly sliced
- 1 bunch asparagus, trimmed and cut into 2-inch pieces
- 1 red bell pepper, thinly sliced
- 1 yellow bell pepper, thinly sliced
- 1 onion, thinly sliced
- 3 cloves garlic, minced
- 1-inch piece ginger, minced
- 1/4 cup coconut aminos
- 2 tbsp olive oil
- Salt and pepper, to taste
- Fresh cilantro or parsley for garnish (optional)

Instructions:

1. Slice the chicken breasts thinly. Trim and cut the asparagus into 2-inch pieces. Thinly slice the red and yellow bell peppers and onion. Mince the garlic and ginger.

2. Heat 1 tablespoon of olive oil in a large skillet or wok over medium-high heat. Add the sliced chicken breasts and stir-fry until fully cooked and no longer pink, about 5-6 minutes. Take out the chicken from the skillet and set aside.

3. In the same skillet, add the remaining 1 tablespoon of olive oil. Add the minced garlic and ginger, and stir-fry for about 1 minute until fragrant. Add the sliced onion and bell peppers, and cook for 3-4 minutes until slightly tender.

4. Return the cooked chicken to the skillet. Add the asparagus pieces. Pour in the coconut aminos and stir everything together. Cook for another 3-4 minutes, or until the asparagus is crisp-tender and everything is heated through. Season with salt and pepper to taste.

5. Garnish with fresh cilantro or parsley if desired. Serve the Chicken and Asparagus Stir-Fry hot, and enjoy!

Nutritional Information:

- **Calories:** 280 kcal
- **Fat:** 10g
- **Carbohydrates:** 12g
- **Protein:** 34g

Beef and Avocado Salad with Lime Cilantro Dressing

Prep Time: 20 minutes | **Cook Time:** 10 minutes | **Total Time:** 30 minutes | **Servings:** 4

Ingredients:

- 1-poundflank steak
- 1 avocado, sliced
- 4 cups mixed salad greens (such as spinach, arugula, and kale)
- 1/2 cup cherry tomatoes, halved
- 1/4 cup red onion, thinly sliced
- 1/4 cup fresh cilantro leaves, chopped
- 2 tbsp olive oil
- 2 tbsp lime juice
- 1 garlic clove, minced
- Salt and pepper, to taste

Instructions:

1. Season the flank steak with salt and pepper. Heat a grill or grill pan over medium-high heat. Grill the steak for about 4-5 minutes per side for medium-rare, or until desired doneness. Remove from heat and let it rest for 5 minutes before slicing thinly against the grain.

2. In a small bowl, whisk together olive oil, lime juice, minced garlic, salt, and pepper to make the lime cilantro dressing.

3. In a large bowl, combine the mixed salad greens, cherry tomatoes, red onion slices, and chopped cilantro. Toss with half of the lime cilantro dressing.

4. Divide the salad mixture among plates. Top each with slices of grilled flank steak and avocado slices. Drizzle with the remaining lime cilantro dressing.

5. Garnish with extra cilantro leaves if desired. Serve the Beef and Avocado Salad immediately.

Nutritional Information:

- **Calories:** 350 kcal
- **Fat:** 22g
- **Carbohydrates:** 10g
- **Protein:** 30g

Zucchini Noodles with Pesto and Grilled Chicken

Prep Time: 15 minutes | **Cook Time:** 15 minutes | **Total Time:** 30 minutes | **Servings:** 4

Ingredients:

- 4 medium zucchinis, spiralized into noodles
- 1-poundchicken breast, grilled and sliced
- 1/2 cup basil pesto (homemade or store-bought)
- 1 cup cherry tomatoes, halved
- 1/4 cup pine nuts, toasted
- 2 tbsp olive oil
- Salt and pepper, to taste
- Fresh basil leaves, for garnish

Instructions:

1. Season the chicken breast with salt and pepper. Grill over medium-high heat until cooked through, about 6-7 minutes per side. Let it rest for a few minutes, then slice into thin strips.

2. In a dry skillet over medium heat, toast the pine nuts until golden and fragrant, stirring frequently to prevent burning. Remove from heat and set aside.

3. Heat olive oil in a large skillet over medium heat. Add the zucchini noodles and sauté for 2-3 minutes until just tender. Season with salt and pepper to taste.

4. Add the grilled chicken slices, cherry tomatoes, and basil pesto to the skillet with the zucchini noodles. Toss gently to combine and heat through for 1-2 minutes.

5. Divide the zucchini noodle mixture among plates. Sprinkle with toasted pine nuts and garnish with fresh basil leaves.

Nutritional Information:

- **Calories:** 380 kcal
- **Fat:** 22g
- **Carbohydrates:** 12g
- **Protein:** 32g

<u>Turkey and Avocado Stuffed Tomatoes</u>

Prep Time: 15 minutes | **Cook Time:** 0 minutes | **Total Time:** 15 minutes | **Servings:** 4

Ingredients:

- 4 large tomatoes
- 1-poundground turkey
- 1 avocado, diced
- 1/4 cup red onion, finely chopped
- 1/4 cup cucumber, diced
- 1/4 cup bell pepper, diced
- 2 tbsp fresh parsley, chopped
- 2 tbsp olive oil
- 1 tbsp lemon juice
- Salt and pepper, to taste
- Fresh basil leaves, for garnish

Instructions:

1. Cut the tops off the tomatoes and carefully scoop out the flesh and seeds to create hollow shells. Set aside.

2. In a skillet over medium heat, cook the ground turkey until fully browned and cooked through, breaking it up into crumbles as it cooks. Drain any excess fat and set aside to cool slightly.

3. In a large bowl, combine the diced avocado, red onion, cucumber, bell pepper, and parsley. Add the cooked ground turkey to the bowl.

4. Drizzle olive oil and lemon juice over the filling mixture. Season with salt and pepper to taste. Mix everything together gently until well combined.

5. Spoon the turkey and avocado mixture into the hollowed-out tomatoes, dividing it evenly among them.

6. Garnish with fresh basil leaves and serve immediately.

Nutritional Information:

- **Calories:** 320 kcal
- **Fat:** 20g
- **Carbohydrates:** 12g
- **Protein:** 25g

Quinoa and Kale Salad with Feta Cheese

Prep Time: 15 minutes | **Cook Time:** 15 minutes | **Total Time:** 30 minutes | **Servings:** 4

Ingredients:

- 1 cup quinoa
- 2 cups water or vegetable broth
- 1 bunch kale, stems removed and leaves chopped
- 1/2 cup cherry tomatoes, halved
- 1/4 cup red onion, finely chopped
- 1/4 cup cucumber, diced
- 1/4 cup feta cheese, crumbled
- 2 tbsp olive oil
- 1 tbsp lemon juice
- 1 tbsp balsamic vinegar
- Salt and pepper, to taste

Instructions:

1. Rinse the quinoa under cold water. In a medium saucepan, bring the water or vegetable broth to a boil. Add the quinoa, reduce heat to low, cover, and simmer for 15 minutes or until all liquid is absorbed. Fluff with a fork and let it cool.

2. In a large bowl, massage the chopped kale with a bit of olive oil for a few minutes until it starts to soften.

3. Add the cooked quinoa, cherry tomatoes, red onion, cucumber, and crumbled feta cheese to the bowl with kale.

4. In a small bowl, whisk together olive oil, lemon juice, balsamic vinegar, salt, and pepper.

5. Pour the dressing over the salad ingredients. Toss gently until everything is well coated with the dressing.

6. Divide the salad into serving bowls and serve immediately.

Nutritional Information:

- **Calories:** 280 kcal
- **Fat:** 12g
- **Carbohydrates:** 33g
- **Protein:** 10g

Grilled Chicken and Broccoli Bowl with Tahini Dressing

Prep Time: 15 minutes | **Cook Time:** 20 minutes | **Total Time:** 35 minutes | **Servings:** 4

Ingredients:

- 1-poundchicken breast, boneless and skinless
- 1-poundbroccoli florets
- 1 tbsp olive oil
- Salt and pepper, to taste
- 1/2 cup quinoa, uncooked
- 1/4 cup tahini

- 2 tbsp lemon juice
- 1 clove garlic, minced
- 2 tbsp water
- 1 tbsp honey or maple syrup (optional, omit for lower sugar)
- Sesame seeds, for garnish (optional)

Instructions:

1. Rinse the quinoa under cold water. In a small saucepan, bring 1 cup of water to a boil. Add the quinoa, reduce heat to low, cover, and simmer for 15 minutes or until all liquid is absorbed. Fluff with a fork and set aside.
2. Preheat grill or grill pan over medium-high heat. Season chicken breasts with salt and pepper.
3. Grill chicken for about 6-7 minutes per side, or until fully cooked (internal temperature of 165°F or 74°C). Remove from grill and let rest for 5 minutes before slicing.
4. Toss broccoli florets with olive oil, salt, and pepper. Grill for 5-7 minutes, turning occasionally, until tender and lightly charred. Remove from grill.
5. In a small bowl, whisk together tahini, lemon juice, minced garlic, water, and honey or maple syrup (if using), until smooth and creamy. Adjust consistency with more water if needed.
6. Divide cooked quinoa, grilled chicken slices, and grilled broccoli among serving bowls.
7. Drizzle tahini dressing over each bowl.
8. Garnish with sesame seeds if desired.
9. Serve immediately and enjoy!

Nutritional Information:

- **Calories:** 380 kcal
- **Fat:** 18g
- **Protein:** 34g

Shrimp and Spinach Salad with Lemon Garlic Dressing

Prep Time: 15 minutes | **Cook Time:** 10 minutes | **Total Time:** 25 minutes | **Servings:** 4

Ingredients:

- 1-poundshrimp, peeled and deveined
- 8 cups fresh spinach leaves
- 1 cup cherry tomatoes, halved
- 1/2 red onion, thinly sliced
- 1 avocado, sliced
- 1/4 cup feta cheese, crumbled (optional)
- 2 tbsp olive oil
- 2 cloves garlic, minced
- Zest and juice of 1 lemon
- Salt and pepper, to taste

Instructions:

1. In a large skillet, heat 1 tablespoon of olive oil over medium-high heat. Add minced garlic and sauté until fragrant.

2. Add shrimp to the skillet and cook for about 2-3 minutes per side, until pink and cooked through. Season with salt and pepper. Remove from heat and set aside.

3. In a small bowl, whisk together the remaining olive oil, lemon zest, lemon juice, and a pinch of salt and pepper to taste. Set aside.

4. In a large bowl, combine spinach leaves, cherry tomatoes, sliced red onion, avocado slices, and crumbled feta cheese (if using).

5. Add the cooked shrimp to the salad.

6. Drizzle the lemon garlic dressing over the salad and gently toss to combine.

7. Serve immediately, garnished with additional lemon zest if desired.

Nutritional Information:

- **Calories:** 320 kcal
- **Fat:** 18g
- **Carbohydrates:** 14g
- **Protein:** 28g

Chapter 5: Fiber-Rich Dinners

Baked Salmon with Quinoa and Asparagus

Prep Time: 15 minutes | **Cook Time:** 20 minutes | **Servings:** 4

Ingredients:

- 4 salmon fillets (about 4 ounces each)
- 1 cup quinoa
- 1 bunch asparagus, trimmed
- 1 lemon, thinly sliced
- 2 tablespoons olive oil
- 2 cloves garlic, minced
- 1 teaspoon dried thyme
- Salt and pepper, to taste
- Fresh parsley, for garnish

Instructions:

1. Preheat the oven to 400°F (200°C).

2. Rinse the quinoa under cold water. In a medium saucepan, bring 2 cups of water to a boil. Add the quinoa, reduce heat to low, cover, and simmer for 15 minutes or until all water is absorbed. Remove from heat and let it sit covered for 5 minutes. Fluff with a fork.

3. Place the salmon fillets on a baking sheet lined with parchment paper. Arrange the asparagus around the salmon. Drizzle olive oil over the salmon and asparagus. Season with minced garlic, dried thyme, salt, and pepper. Place lemon slices on top of each salmon fillet.

4. Transfer the baking sheet to the oven and bake for 15-20 minutes, or until the salmon is cooked through and flakes easily with a fork.

5. Divide the quinoa among plates. Top with baked salmon fillets and roasted asparagus. Garnish with fresh parsley and serve hot.

Nutritional Information (per serving):

- **Calories:** 380 kcal
- **Fat:** 18g
- **Carbohydrates:** 22g
- **Protein:** 30g

Stuffed Bell Peppers with Ground Turkey and Black Beans

Prep Time: 20 minutes | **Cook Time:** 40 minutes | **Servings:** 4

Ingredients:

- 4 large bell peppers, any color
- 1 pound lean ground turkey
- 1 cup cooked quinoa
- 1 can (15 ounces) black beans, drained and rinsed
- 1 cup diced tomatoes
- 1 cup chopped spinach
- 1/2 cup diced onion
- 2 cloves garlic, minced
- 1 teaspoon ground cumin
- 1 teaspoon chili powder
- Salt and pepper, to taste
- 1/2 cup shredded mozzarella cheese (optional)
- Fresh cilantro, for garnish

Instructions:

1. Preheat the oven to 375°F (190°C).
2. Cut the tops off the bell peppers and remove seeds and membranes. Place them upright in a baking dish.
3. In a large skillet, cook ground turkey over medium heat until no longer pink, breaking it apart with a spoon as it cooks.
4. Add diced onion and minced garlic to the skillet with the turkey. Cook for 2-3 minutes until onion is translucent. Stir in cooked quinoa, black beans, diced tomatoes, chopped spinach, ground cumin, chili powder, salt, and pepper. Cook for another 5 minutes until everything is heated through and well combined.
5. Spoon the turkey and quinoa mixture evenly into the bell peppers. If using, sprinkle shredded mozzarella cheese on top.
6. Cover the baking dish with foil and bake for 30 minutes. Take out the foil and bake for an additional 10 minutes, or until the peppers are tender and cheese is melted and bubbly.
7. Remove from oven and let cool slightly. Garnish with fresh cilantro before serving.

Nutritional Information (per serving):

- **Calories:** 380 kcal
- **Fat:** 12g
- **Carbohydrates:** 35g
- **Protein:** 30g

Zucchini Lasagna with Ground Beef

Prep Time: 30 minutes | **Cook Time:** 45 minutes | **Servings:** 6

Ingredients:

- 2 large zucchinis, sliced lengthwise into thin strips
- 1 pound lean ground beef
- 1 onion, finely chopped
- 3 cloves garlic, minced
- 1 bell pepper, diced
- 1 can (15 ounces) crushed tomatoes
- 1 can (6 ounces) tomato paste
- 1 tablespoon olive oil
- 1 teaspoon dried oregano
- 1 teaspoon dried basil
- Salt and pepper, to taste
- 1 cup part-skim ricotta cheese
- 1 cup shredded mozzarella cheese
- Fresh basil, for garnish

Instructions:

1. Preheat the oven to 375°F (190°C).

2. Slice the zucchinis lengthwise into thin strips using a mandoline slicer or a sharp knife. Lay them on paper towels and sprinkle with salt to draw out moisture.

3. In a large skillet, heat olive oil over medium heat. Add chopped onion, minced garlic, and diced bell pepper. Cook for 5 minutes until vegetables are softened. Add ground beef and cook until browned. Drain any excess fat.

4. Stir in crushed tomatoes, tomato paste, dried oregano, dried basil, salt, and pepper to the skillet with the ground beef mixture. Simmer for 10 minutes, stirring occasionally.

5. In a 9x13 inch baking dish, spread a thin layer of the meat sauce. Layer zucchini strips over the sauce. Spread half of the ricotta cheese over the zucchini, then spread half of the remaining meat sauce. Repeat with another layer of zucchini, remaining ricotta cheese, and remaining meat sauce. Top with shredded mozzarella cheese.

6. Cover the baking dish with foil and bake for 30 minutes. Take out the foil and bake for an additional 15 minutes, or until the cheese is melted and bubbly.

7. Remove from oven and let it cool slightly. Garnish with fresh basil before serving.

Nutritional Information (per serving):

- **Calories:** 360 kcal
- **Fat:** 15g
- **Carbohydrates:** 15g
- **Protein:** 35g

Baked Cod with Spinach and Brown Rice

Prep Time: 15 minutes | **Cook Time:** 25 minutes | **Servings:** 4

Ingredients:

- 4 cod fillets (about 6 ounces each)
- 1 cup brown rice, uncooked
- 2 cups fresh spinach leaves
- 1 lemon, thinly sliced
- 2 tablespoons olive oil
- 2 cloves garlic, minced
- 1 teaspoon dried dill
- Salt and pepper, to taste
- Fresh parsley, for garnish

Instructions:

1. Preheat the oven to 400°F (200°C).

2. In a medium saucepan, bring 2 cups of water to a boil. Add the brown rice, reduce heat to low, cover, and simmer for 20-25 minutes or until rice is tender and water is absorbed. Fluff with a fork.

3. Place the cod fillets in a baking dish lined with parchment paper. Arrange spinach leaves around the cod. Drizzle olive oil over the cod and spinach. Season with minced garlic, dried dill, salt, and pepper. Place lemon slices on top of each cod fillet.

4. Transfer the baking dish to the oven and bake for 15-20 minutes, or until the cod is cooked through and flakes easily with a fork.

5. Divide the brown rice among plates. Top with baked cod fillets and spinach. Garnish with fresh parsley and serve hot.

Nutritional Information (per serving):

- **Calories:** 380 kcal
- **Fat:** 12g
- **Carbohydrates:** 30g
- **Protein:** 35g

<u>Chickpea and Vegetable Curry</u>

Prep Time: 15 minutes | **Cook Time:** 30 minutes | **Servings:** 4

Ingredients:

- 1 tablespoon olive oil
- 1 onion, finely chopped
- 3 cloves garlic, minced
- 1 tablespoon fresh ginger, minced
- 1 bell pepper, diced
- 1 zucchini, diced
- 1 carrot, diced

- 1 can (15 ounces) chickpeas, drained and rinsed
- 1 can (14 ounces) coconut milk
- 1 cup vegetable broth
- 2 tablespoons curry powder
- 1 teaspoon ground turmeric
- Salt and pepper, to taste
- Fresh cilantro, for garnish

Instructions:

1. In a large skillet or pot, heat olive oil over medium heat.

2. Add chopped onion, minced garlic, and minced ginger. Cook for 3-4 minutes until onions are translucent and fragrant.

3. Stir in diced bell pepper, zucchini, and carrot. Cook for 5 minutes until vegetables begin to soften.

4. Add drained chickpeas, coconut milk, vegetable broth, curry powder, ground turmeric, salt, and pepper. Stir adequately to combine.

5. Bring the mixture to a boil, then reduce heat to low. Cover and simmer for 15-20 minutes, stirring occasionally, until vegetables are tender and flavors are blended.

6. Remove from heat and let it sit for a few minutes. Serve hot, garnished with fresh cilantro.

Nutritional Information (per serving):

- **Calories:** 380 kcal
- **Fat:** 22g
- **Carbohydrates:** 38g
- **Protein:** 10g

Grilled Shrimp with Cauliflower Rice Pilaf

Prep Time: 15 minutes | **Cook Time:** 20 minutes | **Servings:** 4

Ingredients:

- 1 pound large shrimp, peeled and deveined
- 1 head cauliflower, grated into rice-like texture
- 1 red bell pepper, diced
- 1 onion, finely chopped
- 2 cloves garlic, minced
- 1 tablespoon olive oil
- 1 teaspoon ground cumin
- 1 teaspoon paprika
- Salt and pepper, to taste
- Fresh parsley, for garnish

Instructions:

1. Preheat the grill to medium-high heat.

2. In a bowl, toss the shrimp with olive oil, ground cumin, paprika, salt, and pepper until evenly coated. Set aside.

3. Heat olive oil in a large skillet over medium heat. Add chopped onion and minced garlic, sauté until softened and fragrant, about 3-4 minutes.

4. Add diced red bell pepper and continue to cook for another 3-4 minutes until peppers are tender.

5. Stir in grated cauliflower rice, season with salt and pepper to taste. Cook for about 5-7 minutes until cauliflower is tender but still has a slight crunch.

6. Place seasoned shrimp on the preheated grill. Cook for 2-3 minutes per side, or until shrimp are pink and opaque.

7. Divide the cauliflower rice pilaf among plates. Top with grilled shrimp and garnish with fresh parsley.

Nutritional Information (per serving):

- **Calories:** 280 kcal
- **Fat:** 10g
- **Carbohydrates:** 15g
- **Protein:** 30g

Tofu and Vegetable Stir-Fry with Brown Rice

Prep Time: 15 minutes | **Cook Time:** 20 minutes | **Servings:** 4

Ingredients:

- 1 block (14 oz) firm tofu, pressed and cubed
- 2 cups cooked brown rice
- 1 red bell pepper, thinly sliced
- 1 yellow bell pepper, thinly sliced
- 1 cup snap peas, trimmed
- 1 cup broccoli florets
- 1 carrot, julienned
- 2 cloves garlic, minced
- 1 tablespoon ginger, minced
- 2 tablespoons low-sodium soy sauce
- 1 tablespoon hoisin sauce
- 1 tablespoon sesame oil
- 2 tablespoons olive oil, divided
- Salt and pepper, to taste
- Fresh cilantro or green onions, for garnish

Instructions:

1. Press the tofu to remove excess moisture. Cut into cubes.

2. In a large skillet or wok, heat 1 tablespoon of olive oil over medium-high heat. Add tofu cubes and cook until golden brown on all sides, about 5-7 minutes. Remove tofu from skillet and set aside.

3. In the same skillet or wok, add the remaining olive oil. Add minced garlic and ginger, sauté for about 1 minute until fragrant.

4. Add sliced red and yellow bell peppers, snap peas, broccoli florets, and julienned carrot. Stir-fry for 5-7 minutes until vegetables are tender-crisp.

5. Return the tofu to the skillet with the stir-fried vegetables.

6. In a small bowl, mix together low-sodium soy sauce, hoisin sauce, and sesame oil. Pour the sauce over the tofu and vegetables. Stir to combine and cook for another 2-3 minutes to heat through.

7. Divide the cooked brown rice among plates. Top with tofu and vegetable stir-fry. Garnish with fresh cilantro or green onions.

Nutritional Information (per serving):

- **Calories:** 320 kcal
- **Fat:** 15g
- **Carbohydrates:** 30g
- **Protein:** 18g

Baked Chicken with Broccoli and Quinoa

Prep Time: 15 minutes | **Cook Time:** 30 minutes | **Servings:** 4

Ingredients:

- 4 boneless, skinless chicken breasts
- 1 cup quinoa, rinsed
- 2 cups chicken broth
- 2 cups broccoli florets
- 1 red bell pepper, diced
- 1 onion, diced
- 2 cloves garlic, minced
- 1 tablespoon olive oil
- 1 teaspoon paprika
- 1 teaspoon dried thyme
- Salt and pepper, to taste
- Fresh parsley, for garnish

Instructions:

1. Preheat the oven to 400°F (200°C).
2. Season the chicken breasts with paprika, dried thyme, salt, and pepper on both sides.
3. In a medium saucepan, heat olive oil over medium heat. Add diced onion and garlic, sauté until softened.
4. Add rinsed quinoa and toast for 2-3 minutes.
5. Pour in chicken broth and bring to a boil. Reduce heat, cover, and simmer for 15 minutes or until quinoa is cooked and liquid is absorbed.
6. In a separate skillet, heat olive oil over medium heat. Add diced red bell pepper and broccoli florets. Sauté for 5-7 minutes until vegetables are tender-crisp.
7. Place seasoned chicken breasts on a baking sheet lined with parchment paper or greased lightly. Bake in the preheated oven for 20-25 minutes until chicken is cooked through and reaches an internal temperature of 165°F (75°C).
8. Divide cooked quinoa among plates. Top with baked chicken breasts and sautéed vegetables.
9. Garnish with fresh parsley.

Nutritional Information (per serving):

- **Calories:** 380 kcal
- **Fat:** 10g
- **Carbohydrates:** 35g
- **Protein:** 35g

Stuffed Eggplant with Ground Lamb and Lentils

Prep Time: 20 minutes | **Cook Time:** 50 minutes | **Servings:** 4

Ingredients:

- 2 large eggplants
- 250g lean ground lamb
- 1/2 cup brown lentils, cooked
- 1 onion, finely chopped
- 2 cloves garlic, minced
- 1 red bell pepper, diced
- 1 teaspoon ground cumin
- 1 teaspoon ground coriander
- 1/2 teaspoon ground cinnamon
- Salt and pepper, to taste
- 2 tablespoons olive oil
- 1/4 cup chopped fresh parsley
- 1/4 cup chopped fresh mint
- 1/4 cup crumbled feta cheese (optional, for garnish)

Instructions:

1. Preheat the oven to 400°F (200°C).
2. Cut each eggplant in half lengthwise. Scoop out the flesh, leaving about a 1/2-inch thick shell. Chop the eggplant flesh and set aside.
3. Heat 1 tablespoon of olive oil in a large skillet over medium heat. Add chopped onion and cook until softened, about 5 minutes.
4. Add minced garlic, diced red bell pepper, and chopped eggplant flesh. Cook for another 5-7 minutes until vegetables are tender.
5. Push vegetables to the side of the skillet and add ground lamb. Cook until browned, breaking it up with a spoon as it cooks.
6. Stir in ground cumin, ground coriander, ground cinnamon, salt, and pepper. Cook for 1-2 minutes until fragrant.
7. Stir in cooked lentils, chopped fresh parsley, and chopped fresh mint into the lamb mixture. Remove from heat.
8. Brush the eggplant shells with the remaining olive oil and season with salt and pepper. Place them on a baking sheet.
9. Spoon the lamb and lentil mixture evenly into the eggplant shells, pressing gently to pack.
10. Cover the baking dish with foil and bake in the preheated oven for 30 minutes. Remove foil and bake for an additional 10 minutes until eggplant shells are tender.
11. Remove stuffed eggplants from the oven and let them cool slightly before serving.
12. Garnish with crumbled feta cheese, if desired.

Nutritional Information (per serving):

- **Calories:** 380 kcal
- **Fat:** 20g
- **Carbohydrates:** 25g
- **Protein:** 28g

Roasted Vegetable and Chickpea Bowl

Prep Time: 15 minutes | **Cook Time:** 30 minutes | **Servings:** 4

Ingredients:

- 1 medium sweet potato, peeled and diced
- 1 small head of cauliflower, cut into florets
- 1 red bell pepper, seeded and sliced
- 1 small red onion, sliced
- 1 can (15 oz) chickpeas, drained and rinsed
- 2 tablespoons olive oil
- 1 teaspoon ground cumin
- 1 teaspoon paprika
- Salt and pepper, to taste
- 4 cups mixed greens (spinach, arugula, or kale)
- 1 avocado, sliced
- 1/4 cup chopped fresh parsley or cilantro
- 2 tablespoons tahini (optional, for drizzling)

Instructions:

1. Preheat the oven to 400°F (200°C).

2. In a large bowl, toss diced sweet potato, cauliflower florets, sliced red bell pepper, red onion, and chickpeas with olive oil, ground cumin, paprika, salt, and pepper until evenly coated.

3. Spread the vegetables and chickpeas in a single layer on a baking sheet. Roast in the preheated oven for 25-30 minutes, stirring halfway through, until vegetables are tender and lightly browned.

4. While the vegetables are roasting, divide mixed greens among serving bowls. Top with sliced avocado.

5. Once roasted, divide the roasted vegetable and chickpea mixture among the serving bowls over the mixed greens and avocado.

6. Sprinkle chopped fresh parsley or cilantro over each bowl.

7. Drizzle with tahini, if using, before serving.

Nutritional Information (per serving):

- **Calories:** 380 kcal
- **Fat:** 20g
- **Carbohydrates:** 42g
- **Protein:** 12g

Grilled Pork Chops with Apple and Brussels Sprout Slaw

Prep Time: 20 minutes | **Cook Time:** 15 minutes | **Servings:** 4

Ingredients:

- 4 boneless pork chops
- 2 tablespoons olive oil
- Salt and pepper, to taste
- 1 large apple, cored and thinly sliced
- 1 cup shredded Brussels sprouts
- 1/4 cup chopped walnuts
- 2 tablespoons apple cider vinegar
- 1 tablespoon Dijon mustard
- 1 tablespoon honey (optional)
- 2 tablespoons chopped fresh parsley or cilantro

Instructions:

1. Preheat the grill to medium-high heat.
2. Rub pork chops with olive oil and season with salt and pepper.
3. Grill the pork chops for about 5-7 minutes per side, or until internal temperature reaches 145°F (63°C). Remove from grill and let rest for a few minutes.
4. In a large bowl, combine apple slices, shredded Brussels sprouts, chopped walnuts, apple cider vinegar, Dijon mustard, and honey (if using). Toss until well combined. Season with salt and pepper to taste.
5. Divide the apple and Brussels sprout slaw among serving plates.
6. Place grilled pork chops on top of the slaw.
7. Garnish with chopped fresh parsley or cilantro.

Nutritional Information (per serving):

- **Calories:** 320 kcal
- **Fat:** 18g
- **Carbohydrates:** 12g
- **Protein:** 28g

Baked Haddock with Spinach and Quinoa

Prep Time: 15 minutes | **Cook Time:** 25 minutes | **Servings:** 4

Ingredients:

- 4 haddock fillets (about 6 ounces each)
- 1 cup quinoa, rinsed
- 2 cups low-sodium vegetable broth or water
- 1 tablespoon olive oil
- 2 cloves garlic, minced
- 6 cups fresh spinach
- Juice of 1 lemon
- Salt and pepper, to taste
- Fresh parsley, chopped (for garnish)

Instructions:

1. Preheat the oven to 375°F (190°C).

2. In a medium saucepan, bring the vegetable broth or water to a boil. Add quinoa, reduce heat to low, cover, and simmer for about 15 minutes or until quinoa is cooked and liquid is absorbed. Fluff with a fork.

3. Place haddock fillets on a baking sheet lined with parchment paper or lightly greased. Season with salt and pepper.

4. Bake in the preheated oven for 12-15 minutes, or until the fish flakes easily with a fork.

5. While the haddock is baking, heat olive oil in a large skillet over medium heat. Add minced garlic and cook for about 1 minute, until fragrant.

6. Add spinach to the skillet in batches, stirring until wilted. Add lemon juice and season with salt and pepper to taste.

7. To serve, divide quinoa among plates, top with spinach, and place baked haddock fillets on top. Garnish with chopped fresh parsley.

Nutritional Information (per serving):

- **Calories:** 320 kcal
- **Fat:** 9g
- **Carbohydrates:** 27g
- **Protein:** 32g

Black Bean and Sweet Potato Enchiladas

Prep Time: 30 minutes | **Cook Time:** 30 minutes | **Servings:** 4

Ingredients:

- 1 tablespoon olive oil
- 1 small onion, diced
- 2 cloves garlic, minced
- 1 teaspoon ground cumin
- 1 teaspoon chili powder
- 1 can (15 ounces) black beans, drained and rinsed
- 2 cups cooked sweet potatoes, mashed
- 1 cup corn kernels (fresh or frozen)
- 1/2 cup chopped fresh cilantro
- Juice of 1 lime
- Salt and pepper, to taste
- 8 whole wheat or corn tortillas
- 1 cup enchilada sauce (store-bought or homemade)
- 1 cup shredded Monterey Jack cheese (optional, omit for dairy-free)
- Chopped green onions, for garnish

Instructions:

1. Preheat the oven to 375°F (190°C). Lightly grease a 9x13-inch baking dish.

2. Heat olive oil in a large skillet over medium heat. Add diced onion and cook until translucent, about 5 minutes. Add minced garlic, ground cumin, and chili powder. Cook for 1 minute until fragrant.

3. Stir in black beans, mashed sweet potatoes, corn kernels, chopped cilantro, and lime juice. Season with salt and pepper to taste. Cook for 5 minutes until heated through.

4. Spread about 1/4 cup of enchilada sauce in the bottom of the prepared baking dish.

5. Place a tortilla on a flat surface. Spoon about 1/3 cup of the filling mixture down the center of the tortilla. Roll up tightly and place seam side down in the baking dish. Repeat with remaining tortillas and filling.

6. Pour remaining enchilada sauce over the assembled enchiladas. If using cheese, sprinkle it evenly over the top.

7. Cover the baking dish with aluminum foil and bake in the preheated oven for 20 minutes. Take out the foil and bake for an additional 10 minutes, until the enchiladas are heated through and the cheese is melted and bubbly.

8. Remove from the oven and let cool slightly before serving. Garnish with chopped green onions if desired.

Nutritional Information (per serving):

- **Calories:** 420 kcal
- **Fat:** 12g
- **Carbohydrates:** 62g
- **Protein:** 16g

Grilled Steak with Asparagus and Wild Rice

Prep Time: 15 minutes | **Cook Time:** 20 minutes | **Servings:** 4

Ingredients:

- 4 beef sirloin steaks, about 6 ounces each
- Salt and pepper, to taste
- 1 bunch asparagus, tough ends trimmed
- 1 tablespoon olive oil
- 2 cups cooked wild rice
- 2 tablespoons chopped fresh parsley
- Lemon wedges, for serving

Instructions:

1. Preheat the grill to medium-high heat.

2. Season the steaks generously with salt and pepper on both sides.

3. Grill the steaks for 4-5 minutes per side for medium-rare, or to your desired doneness. Remove from the grill and let rest for 5 minutes.

4. While the steaks are resting, toss the trimmed asparagus with olive oil, salt, and pepper.

5. Grill the asparagus on the preheated grill for about 5-7 minutes, turning occasionally, until tender and lightly charred. Remove from the grill.

6. Divide the cooked wild rice among plates. Top with grilled steaks and asparagus. Sprinkle with chopped parsley. Serve with lemon wedges on the side.

Nutritional Information (per serving):

- **Calories:** 480 kcal
- **Fat:** 20g
- **Carbohydrates:** 25g
- **Protein:** 48g

<u>**Veggie and Quinoa Stuffed Bell Peppers**</u>

Prep Time: 20 minutes | **Cook Time:** 40 minutes | **Servings:** 4

Ingredients:

- 4 large bell peppers, any color
- 1 cup quinoa, rinsed
- 2 cups vegetable broth
- 1 tablespoon olive oil
- 1 onion, finely chopped
- 2 cloves garlic, minced
- 1 zucchini, diced
- 1 carrot, diced
- 1 cup cherry tomatoes, halved
- 1 teaspoon dried oregano
- 1 teaspoon dried basil
- Salt and pepper, to taste
- 1/2 cup grated mozzarella cheese (optional)
- Fresh parsley or basil, chopped, for garnish

Instructions:

1. Preheat the oven to 375°F (190°C).

2. Cut the tops off the bell peppers and take out the seeds and membranes. Place them upright in a baking dish.

3. In a saucepan, combine quinoa and vegetable broth. Bring to a boil, then reduce heat to low, cover, and simmer for 15 minutes or until quinoa is cooked and liquid is absorbed.

4. In a large skillet, heat olive oil over medium heat. Add onion and garlic, sauté until softened, about 3 minutes.

5. Add diced zucchini, carrot, cherry tomatoes, dried oregano, dried basil, salt, and pepper. Cook for 5-7 minutes until vegetables are tender.

6. Stir cooked quinoa into the skillet with the sautéed vegetables. Adjust seasoning if needed.

7. Spoon the quinoa and vegetable mixture evenly into the prepared bell peppers. If using cheese, sprinkle grated mozzarella on top of each stuffed pepper.

8. Cover the baking dish with foil and bake in the preheated oven for 25-30 minutes, or until the peppers are tender.

9. Remove from the oven and garnish with fresh chopped parsley or basil. Serve hot.

Nutritional Information (per serving):

- **Calories:** 340 kcal
- **Fat:** 9g
- **Carbohydrates:** 54g
- **Protein:** 12g

Chicken and Vegetable Skewers with Brown Rice

Prep Time: 20 minutes | **Cook Time:** 20 minutes | **Servings:** 4

Ingredients:

- 1-poundchicken breast, cut into 1-inch cubes
- 2 bell peppers (any color), cut into 1-inch pieces
- 1 zucchini, sliced into rounds
- 1 red onion, cut into wedges
- 8-10 cherry tomatoes
- 1 cup brown rice
- 2 cups water or chicken broth
- 2 tablespoons olive oil
- 1 teaspoon dried oregano
- 1 teaspoon dried basil
- Salt and pepper, to taste
- Wooden skewers, soaked in water for 30 minutes

Instructions:

1. In a saucepan, bring 2 cups of water or chicken broth to a boil. Add brown rice, reduce heat to low, cover, and simmer for 15-20 minutes or until rice is tender and liquid is absorbed.

2. Preheat the grill or grill pan over medium-high heat.

3. Thread the chicken pieces, bell peppers, zucchini slices, red onion wedges, and cherry tomatoes alternately onto the soaked wooden skewers.

4. Brush the skewers with olive oil and sprinkle with dried oregano, dried basil, salt, and pepper.

5. Grill the skewers for about 10 minutes, turning occasionally, until the chicken is cooked through and vegetables are tender and slightly charred.

6. Serve the chicken and vegetable skewers hot with the cooked brown rice.

Nutritional Information (per serving):

- **Calories:** 380 kcal
- **Fat:** 12g
- **Carbohydrates:** 38g
- **Protein:** 30g

Eggplant and Lentil Moussaka

Prep Time: 30 minutes | **Cook Time:** 1 hour | **Servings:** 6

Ingredients:

- 2 large eggplants, sliced lengthwise into 1/2-inch slices
- 1 cup green lentils, rinsed
- 2 cups vegetable broth or water
- 1 onion, finely chopped
- 3 cloves garlic, minced
- 1 red bell pepper, diced
- 1 zucchini, diced
- 1 carrot, diced
- 1 teaspoon dried oregano
- 1 teaspoon dried basil
- 1/2 teaspoon ground cinnamon
- Salt and pepper, to taste
- 1 can (14 oz) diced tomatoes
- 2 tablespoons tomato paste
- 2 tablespoons olive oil
- 1/4 cup grated Parmesan cheese (optional)
- Fresh parsley, chopped, for garnish

Instructions:

1. Preheat the oven to 400°F (200°C). Place the eggplant slices on a baking sheet lined with parchment paper. Brush both sides with olive oil and sprinkle with salt. Bake for 15-20 minutes until tender. Remove from oven and set aside.
2. In a medium saucepan, bring the vegetable broth or water to a boil. Add the rinsed lentils, reduce heat to low, cover, and simmer for 15-20 minutes or until lentils are tender and liquid is absorbed. Remove from heat and set aside.
3. In a large skillet or frying pan, heat olive oil over medium heat. Add the chopped onion and garlic, sauté until softened and fragrant, about 3-4 minutes.
4. Add the diced red bell pepper, zucchini, and carrot. Cook for another 5 minutes until vegetables are slightly tender.
5. Stir in dried oregano, dried basil, ground cinnamon, salt, and pepper. Add diced tomatoes and tomato paste. Cook for 10 minutes until sauce thickens slightly.
6. In a greased 9x13-inch baking dish, layer half of the baked eggplant slices at the bottom.
7. Spread half of the cooked lentils over the eggplant layer.
8. Pour half of the vegetable sauce evenly over the lentils.
9. Repeat with another layer of the remaining eggplant slices, lentils, and vegetable sauce.
10. Cover the baking dish with aluminum foil and bake in the preheated oven at 375°F (190°C) for 30 minutes.
11. Take out the foil, sprinkle grated Parmesan cheese (if using) over the top, and bake uncovered for another 10 minutes until cheese is melted and lightly browned.
12. Garnish with chopped fresh parsley before serving. Serve hot.

Nutritional Information (per serving):

- **Calories:** 320 kcal
- **Fat:** 8g
- **Carbohydrates:** 47g
- **Protein:** 15g

Chapter 6: Low-Carb Snacks

Almond and Coconut Energy Balls

Prep Time: 15 minutes | **Cook Time:** No cook | **Number of Servings:** 12 balls

Ingredients:

- 1 cup almonds, finely ground
- 1/2 cup shredded coconut
- 1/4 cup almond butter
- 1/4 cup honey
- 1 teaspoon vanilla extract
- 1/4 teaspoon sea salt
- Additional shredded coconut for rolling

Instructions:

1. In a food processor, pulse the almonds until finely ground.
2. Add the shredded coconut, almond butter, honey, vanilla extract, and sea salt. Process until the mixture comes together and is sticky.
3. Roll the mixture into tablespoon-sized balls.
4. Roll each ball in shredded coconut to coat.
5. Refrigerate for at least 30 minutes before serving.

Nutritional Information:

- **Calories:** 130 kcal
- **Fat:** 9g
- **Carbohydrates:** 10g
- **Protein:** 4g

Celery Sticks with Almond Butter

Prep Time: 10 minutes | **Cook Time:** No cook | **Number of Servings:** 4 servings

Ingredients:

- 4 celery stalks, washed and trimmed
- 1/2 cup almond butter
- 2 tablespoons unsweetened shredded coconut
- 2 tablespoons chopped almonds
- 1 tablespoon chia seeds
- 1 tablespoon honey (optional, for drizzling)

Instructions:

1. Cut each celery stalk into halves or thirds, depending on size.
2. Spread almond butter into the celery stalks.
3. Sprinkle shredded coconut, chopped almonds, and chia seeds over the almond butter.
4. Drizzle honey over the top, if desired.
5. Serve immediately.

Nutritional Information:

- **Calories:** 230 kcal
- **Fat:** 18g
- **Carbohydrates:** 11g
- **Protein:** 7g

Cheese and Turkey Roll-Ups

Prep Time: 10 minutes | **Cook Time:** No cook | **Number of Servings:** 4 servings

Ingredients:

- 4 slices low-sodium turkey breast
- 4 slices reduced-fat cheese (such as cheddar or Swiss)
- 1/2 avocado, sliced
- 1 cup baby spinach leaves
- 1 tablespoon olive oil
- 1 tablespoon balsamic vinegar
- Salt and pepper to taste

Instructions:

1. Lay out the turkey slices on a clean surface.
2. Place one slice of cheese on each turkey slice.
3. Divide the avocado slices and baby spinach evenly among the turkey slices.
4. Drizzle each with olive oil and balsamic vinegar.
5. Season with salt and pepper to taste.
6. Roll up each turkey slice tightly and secure with toothpicks if needed.
7. Serve immediately or refrigerate until ready to serve.

Nutritional Information:

- **Calories:** 240 kcal
- **Fat:** 15g
- **Carbohydrates:** 6g
- **Protein:** 20g

Cucumber Slices with Hummus

Prep Time: 10 minutes | **Cook Time:** No cook | **Number of Servings:** 4 servings

Ingredients:

- 1 large cucumber, sliced into rounds
- 1/2 cup hummus (homemade or store-bought)
- 1 tablespoon olive oil
- 1 tablespoon lemon juice
- 1/4 teaspoon ground cumin
- Salt and pepper to taste
- Fresh parsley or dill for garnish (optional)

Instructions:

1. Arrange the cucumber slices on a serving platter.
2. In a small bowl, whisk together olive oil, lemon juice, ground cumin, salt, and pepper.
3. Drizzle the olive oil mixture over the cucumber slices.
4. Spoon a dollop of hummus onto each cucumber slice.
5. Garnish with fresh parsley or dill, if desired.
6. Serve immediately.

Nutritional Information:

- **Calories:** 130 kcal
- **Fat:** 9g
- **Carbohydrates:** 9g
- **Protein:** 4g

Greek Yogurt with Blueberries

Prep Time: 5 minutes | **Cook Time:** No cook | **Number of Servings:** 2 servings

Ingredients:

- 1 cup Greek yogurt (plain, unsweetened)
- 1/2 cup fresh blueberries
- 1 tablespoon chopped walnuts
- 1 tablespoon ground flaxseeds
- 1 teaspoon honey (optional, for drizzling)

Instructions:

1. Divide the Greek yogurt evenly between two bowls.
2. Top each bowl of yogurt with fresh blueberries.
3. Sprinkle chopped walnuts and ground flaxseeds over the yogurt and blueberries.
4. Drizzle honey over the top, if desired.
5. Serve immediately.

Nutritional Information:

- **Calories:** 180 kcal
- **Fat:** 8g
- **Carbohydrates:** 15g
- **Protein:** 12g

Mixed Nuts and Seeds

Prep Time: 5 minutes | **Cook Time:** No cook | **Number of Servings:** 4 servings

Ingredients:

- 1/2 cup almonds, unsalted
- 1/2 cup walnuts, unsalted
- 1/4 cup pumpkin seeds
- 1/4 cup sunflower seeds
- 1 tablespoon chia seeds
- 1 tablespoon flaxseeds
- 1/4 teaspoon ground cinnamon
- 1/4 teaspoon sea salt

Instructions:

1. In a mixing bowl, combine almonds, walnuts, pumpkin seeds, sunflower seeds, chia seeds, and flaxseeds.

2. Sprinkle ground cinnamon and sea salt over the nut and seed mixture.

3. Toss gently to combine all ingredients evenly.

4. Serve immediately or store in an airtight container for later use.

Nutritional Information:

- **Calories:** 230 kcal
- **Fat:** 18g
- **Carbohydrates:** 8g
- **Protein:** 9g

Hard-Boiled Eggs with Avocado

Prep Time: 10 minutes | **Cook Time:** 12 minutes | **Number of Servings:** 2 servings

Ingredients:

- 4 large eggs
- 1 ripe avocado
- 1/4 teaspoon sea salt
- 1/4 teaspoon black pepper
- Fresh cilantro or parsley for garnish (optional)

Instructions:

1. Place the eggs in a saucepan and cover with cold water.
2. Bring the water to a boil over medium-high heat.
3. Once boiling, cover the saucepan and remove from heat. Let the eggs sit in the hot water for 10-12 minutes.
4. Drain the hot water and transfer the eggs to a bowl of ice water. Let them cool for a few minutes, then peel and slice each egg in half lengthwise.
5. While the eggs are cooking, cut the avocado in half, take out the pit, and scoop the flesh into a small bowl.
6. Mash the avocado with a fork until smooth. Season with sea salt and black pepper to taste.
7. Arrange the hard-boiled egg halves on a serving plate.
8. Spoon the mashed avocado mixture onto each egg half.
9. Garnish with fresh cilantro or parsley, if desired.
10. Serve immediately as a nutritious and satisfying snack or light meal.

Nutritional Information:

- **Calories:** 215 kcal
- **Fat:** 15g
- **Carbohydrates:** 9g
- **Protein:** 12g

Bell Pepper Strips with Guacamole

Prep Time: 15 minutes | **Cook Time:** 0 minutes | **Number of Servings:** 4 servings

Ingredients:

- 2 large bell peppers (any color), sliced into strips
- 2 ripe avocados
- 1 tomato, diced
- 1/4 cup red onion, finely chopped
- 1 clove garlic, minced
- Juice of 1 lime
- 1/4 teaspoon sea salt
- 1/4 teaspoon black pepper
- Fresh cilantro, chopped, for garnish (optional)

Instructions:

1. Cut the avocados in half, take out the pits, and scoop the flesh into a mixing bowl.

2. Mash the avocado with a fork until smooth or slightly chunky, depending on your preference.

3. Add the diced tomato, chopped red onion, minced garlic, lime juice, sea salt, and black pepper to the bowl. Stir adequately to combine.

4. Wash the bell peppers thoroughly, take out the seeds and stem, and slice them into long strips.

5. Arrange the bell pepper strips on a serving platter.

6. Serve the guacamole alongside the bell pepper strips.

7. Garnish with fresh chopped cilantro, if desired.

8. Serve immediately as a nutritious snack or appetizer.

Nutritional Information:

- **Calories:** 165 kcal
- **Fat:** 13g
- **Carbohydrates:** 13g
- **Protein:** 3g

Turkey and Cheese Lettuce Wraps

Prep Time: 15 minutes | **Cook Time:** 0 minutes | **Number of Servings:** 4 servings

Ingredients:

- 1-poundlean turkey breast, thinly sliced
- 4 large lettuce leaves (such as romaine or butter lettuce)
- 4 slices low-fat cheese (such as Swiss or cheddar)
- 1/2 cup cherry tomatoes, halved
- 1/4 cup red onion, thinly sliced
- 1/4 cup cucumber, thinly sliced
- 1/4 cup bell peppers (any color), thinly sliced
- 1/4 cup avocado, sliced
- 1 tablespoon olive oil
- 1 tablespoon balsamic vinegar
- Salt and pepper, to taste

Instructions:

1. Heat olive oil in a skillet over medium-high heat. Add the turkey breast slices and cook until browned and cooked through, about 3-4 minutes per side. Season with salt and pepper to taste. Remove from heat and set aside.

2. Lay out the lettuce leaves on a clean surface.

3. Place one slice of cheese on each lettuce leaf.

4. Divide the cooked turkey evenly among the lettuce leaves.

5. Top each lettuce wrap with cherry tomatoes, red onion, cucumber, bell peppers, and avocado slices.

6. In a small bowl, whisk together olive oil and balsamic vinegar to make a simple vinaigrette.

7. Drizzle the vinaigrette over the lettuce wraps.

8. Carefully roll up each lettuce leaf to enclose the filling.

9. Secure with toothpicks if needed.

10. Serve immediately.

Nutritional Information:

- **Calories:** 265 kcal
- **Fat:** 12g
- **Carbohydrates:** 8g
- **Protein:** 31g

Almond Flour Crackers with Cheese

Prep Time: 15 minutes | **Cook Time:** 15 minutes | **Number of Servings:** 6 servings

Ingredients:

- 1 1/2 cups almond flour
- 1 tablespoon ground flaxseed
- 1/2 teaspoon baking powder
- 1/2 teaspoon garlic powder
- 1/2 teaspoon onion powder
- 1/4 teaspoon salt
- 1/4 cup grated Parmesan cheese
- 1 large egg
- 2 tablespoons olive oil
- 2 tablespoons water

Instructions:

1. Preheat the oven to 325°F (165°C). Line a baking sheet with parchment paper.

2. In a mixing bowl, combine almond flour, ground flaxseed, baking powder, garlic powder, onion powder, salt, and grated Parmesan cheese.

3. Add the egg, olive oil, and water to the dry ingredients. Mix adequately until a dough forms.

4. Place the dough onto the prepared baking sheet. Cover with another piece of parchment paper.

5. Roll the dough out evenly between the two pieces of parchment paper until it is about 1/8 inch thick.

6. Take out the top parchment paper and use a knife or pizza cutter to cut the dough into squares or rectangles.

7. Bake in the preheated oven for 12-15 minutes, or until the edges are golden brown and crisp.

8. Remove from the oven and allow the crackers to cool completely on the baking sheet. They will crisp up further as they cool.

9. Serve with cheese slices or your preferred dip.

Nutritional Information:

- **Calories:** 210 kcal
- **Fat:** 18g
- **Carbohydrates:** 6g
- **Protein:** 8g

Cherry Tomatoes with Mozzarella Balls

Prep Time: 10 minutes | **Cook Time:** 0 minutes | **Number of Servings:** 4 servings

Ingredients:

- 1-pint cherry tomatoes
- 8 oz mini mozzarella balls (bocconcini), drained
- 1/4 cup fresh basil leaves, torn
- 2 tablespoons extra virgin olive oil
- 1 tablespoon balsamic vinegar
- Salt and pepper, to taste

Instructions:

1. Wash the cherry tomatoes and basil leaves. Drain the mini mozzarella balls.
2. In a large bowl, combine the cherry tomatoes, mini mozzarella balls, and torn basil leaves.
3. Drizzle extra virgin olive oil and balsamic vinegar over the salad ingredients.
4. Season with salt and pepper to taste.
5. Gently toss all ingredients together until evenly combined.
6. Transfer to a serving dish or individual plates.

Nutritional Information:

- **Calories:** 160 kcal
- **Fat:** 12g
- **Carbohydrates:** 5g
- **Protein:** 8g

Sliced Apple with Almond Butter

Prep Time: 5 minutes | **Cook Time:** 0 minutes | **Number of Servings:** 2 servings

Ingredients:

- 1 large apple, thinly sliced

- 4 tablespoons almond butter

- 1 tablespoon chia seeds (optional)

- Cinnamon, for sprinkling

Instructions:

1. Wash and thinly slice the apple.

2. Arrange the apple slices on a serving plate or individual plates.

3. Spread 2 tablespoons of almond butter evenly over the apple slices.

4. Optionally, sprinkle chia seeds over the almond butter.

5. Lightly sprinkle cinnamon over the dish.

6. Serve immediately and enjoy!

Nutritional Information:

- **Calories:** 250 kcal

- **Fat:** 18g

- **Carbohydrates:** 20g

- **Protein:** 7g

Greek Yogurt and Cucumber Dip

Prep Time: 10 minutes | **Cook Time:** 0 minutes | **Number of Servings:** 4 servings

Ingredients:

- 1 cup Greek yogurt
- 1 medium cucumber, grated and excess water squeezed out
- 2 cloves garlic, minced
- 1 tablespoon fresh dill, chopped
- 1 tablespoon fresh lemon juice
- Salt and pepper, to taste
- Olive oil, for drizzling (optional)

Instructions:

1. Grate the cucumber and squeeze out excess water using a clean kitchen towel or paper towels.
2. Mince the garlic cloves.
3. Chop the fresh dill.
4. In a mixing bowl, combine the Greek yogurt, grated cucumber, minced garlic, chopped dill, and fresh lemon juice. Mix adequately.
5. Season the dip with salt and pepper to taste. Adjust seasoning as needed.
6. Transfer the dip to a serving bowl.
7. Optionally, drizzle with a little olive oil before serving.
8. Serve chilled or at room temperature with vegetable sticks or whole grain crackers.

Nutritional Information:

- **Calories:** 60 kcal
- **Fat:** 2g
- **Carbohydrates:** 5g
- **Protein:** 6g

Zucchini Chips with Greek Yogurt Dip

Prep Time: 15 minutes | **Cook Time:** 25 minutes | **Number of Servings:** 4 servings

Ingredients:

- 2 medium zucchinis, sliced into thin rounds
- 1 tablespoon olive oil

- 1/2 teaspoon garlic powder
- 1/2 teaspoon paprika
- Salt and pepper, to taste

For Greek Yogurt Dip:

- 1 cup Greek yogurt
- 1 tablespoon lemon juice
- 1 clove garlic, minced

- 1 tablespoon fresh dill, chopped
- Salt and pepper, to taste

Instructions:

1. Preheat the oven to 425°F (220°C). Line a baking sheet with parchment paper.

2. Slice the zucchinis into thin rounds. Pat them dry with a paper towel to remove excess moisture.

3. In a bowl, toss the zucchini slices with olive oil, garlic powder, paprika, salt, and pepper until evenly coated.

4. Arrange the zucchini slices in a single layer on the prepared baking sheet.

5. Bake in the preheated oven for 20-25 minutes, flipping halfway through, until the chips are golden and crispy.

6. While the zucchini chips are baking, prepare the dip.

7. In a small bowl, mix together Greek yogurt, lemon juice, minced garlic, chopped dill, salt, and pepper. Adjust seasoning to taste.

8. Once the zucchini chips are done, remove from the oven and let them cool slightly.

9. Serve the zucchini chips warm or at room temperature alongside the Greek yogurt dip.

Nutritional Information:

- **Calories:** 120 kcal
- **Fat:** 7g
- **Carbohydrates:** 7g
- **Protein:** 8g

Avocado and Cucumber Sushi Rolls

Prep Time: 30 minutes | **Cook Time:** 0 minutes | **Number of Servings:** 4 servings

Ingredients:

- 4 nori seaweed sheets
- 2 cups cooked sushi rice, cooled
- 1 avocado, thinly sliced
- 1 cucumber, julienned
- 1/2 red bell pepper, julienned
- 1 tablespoon rice vinegar
- 1 tablespoon sesame seeds
- Soy sauce, for serving
- Pickled ginger and wasabi, optional, for serving

Instructions:

1. Cook the sushi rice according to package instructions and let it cool. Mix rice vinegar into the cooled rice.

2. Prepare the avocado by slicing it thinly. Julienne the cucumber and red bell pepper.

3. Place a nori sheet on a bamboo sushi mat (or a clean kitchen towel).

4. Spread an even layer of sushi rice over the nori sheet, leaving about 1 inch of space at the top.

5. Arrange avocado slices, cucumber, and red bell pepper along the center of the rice.

6. Using the bamboo mat, roll the sushi tightly, starting from the bottom edge. Moisten the top edge of the nori with a little water to seal the roll.

7. With a sharp knife, slice each roll into 6-8 pieces. Clean the knife between slices for cleaner cuts.

8. Arrange the sushi rolls on a plate. Sprinkle sesame seeds on top.

9. Serve with soy sauce, and optionally, pickled ginger and wasabi on the side.

Nutritional Information:

- **Calories:** 280 kcal
- **Fat:** 10g
- **Carbohydrates:** 41g
- **Protein:** 6g

Smoked Salmon and Cream Cheese Cucumber Bites

Prep Time: 15 minutes | **Cook Time:** 0 minutes | **Servings:** 12 bites

Ingredients:

- 1 English cucumber
- 4 oz smoked salmon, thinly sliced
- 4 oz cream cheese, softened
- 1 tablespoon fresh dill, chopped
- 1 tablespoon capers, drained and chopped
- Freshly ground black pepper, to taste

Instructions:

1. Wash the cucumber and dill. Pat dry.
2. Chop the fresh dill and capers.
3. Cut the cucumber into 1-inch thick slices.
4. In a small bowl, mix together the softened cream cheese, chopped dill, chopped capers, and freshly ground black pepper.
5. Using a small spoon or knife, scoop out a small indentation in each cucumber slice to create a cup-like shape.
6. Fill each cucumber cup with a generous amount of the cream cheese mixture.
7. Top each cucumber cup with a slice of smoked salmon.
8. Garnish with additional dill or capers if desired.
9. Arrange on a serving platter and serve immediately.

Nutritional Information (per bite):

- **Calories:** 35 kcal
- **Fat:** 2.5 g
- **Carbohydrates:** 1 g
- **Protein:** 2.5 g
- **Cholesterol:** 8 mg

Roasted Chickpeas with Spices

Prep Time: 10 minutes | **Cook Time:** 30 minutes | **Servings:** 4 servings

Ingredients:

- 2 cans (15 oz each) chickpeas (garbanzo beans), drained, rinsed, and patted dry
- 2 tablespoons olive oil
- 1 teaspoon ground cumin
- 1 teaspoon paprika
- 1/2 teaspoon garlic powder
- 1/2 teaspoon onion powder
- 1/2 teaspoon salt
- Freshly ground black pepper, to taste

Instructions:

1. Preheat your oven to 400°F (200°C).

2. Rinse and drain the chickpeas. Pat them dry using a paper towel to remove excess moisture.

3. In a large bowl, toss the chickpeas with olive oil, ground cumin, paprika, garlic powder, onion powder, salt, and freshly ground black pepper until evenly coated.

4. Spread the seasoned chickpeas in a single layer on a baking sheet lined with parchment paper or a silicone baking mat.

5. Roast in the preheated oven for 25-30 minutes, shaking the pan halfway through, until the chickpeas are golden and crispy.

6. Remove from the oven and let cool slightly before serving. Enjoy as a crunchy snack or a topping for salads.

Nutritional Information (per serving):

- **Calories:** 215 kcal
- **Fat:** 8 g
- **Carbohydrates:** 28 g
- **Protein:** 8 g
- **Cholesterol:** 0 mg

Baked Kale Chips

Prep Time: 10 minutes | **Cook Time:** 15 minutes | **Servings:** 4 servings

Ingredients:

- 1 bunch kale (about 10 oz), stems removed and leaves torn into bite-sized pieces
- 1 tablespoon olive oil
- 1/2 teaspoon garlic powder
- 1/2 teaspoon onion powder
- 1/4 teaspoon smoked paprika
- 1/4 teaspoon salt
- Freshly ground black pepper, to taste

Instructions:

1. Preheat your oven to 300°F (150°C).

2. Wash the kale thoroughly and dry completely using a salad spinner or paper towels. Take out the stems and tear the leaves into bite-sized pieces.

3. In a large bowl, drizzle the kale pieces with olive oil. Sprinkle garlic powder, onion powder, smoked paprika, salt, and freshly ground black pepper over the kale. Toss well to coat evenly.

4. Arrange the seasoned kale in a single layer on a baking sheet lined with parchment paper or a silicone baking mat.

5. Bake in the preheated oven for 10-15 minutes, or until the kale is crispy but not burnt. Rotate the baking sheet halfway through baking for even crisping.

6. Remove from the oven and let the kale chips cool on the baking sheet for a few minutes before serving. Enjoy immediately as a healthy snack.

Nutritional Information (per serving):

- **Calories:** 50 kcal
- **Fat:** 3 g
- **Carbohydrates:** 5 g
- **Protein:** 2 g
- **Cholesterol:** 0 mg

Radish and Carrot Sticks with Tzatziki

Prep Time: 15 minutes | **Cook Time:** 0 minutes | **Servings:** 4 servings

Ingredients:

- 1 bunch radishes, washed and trimmed
- 2 large carrots, peeled and cut into sticks
- 1 cup plain Greek yogurt
- 1/2 cucumber, grated and excess moisture squeezed out
- 1 clove garlic, minced
- 1 tablespoon fresh dill, chopped
- 1 tablespoon fresh lemon juice
- Salt and freshly ground black pepper, to taste

Instructions:

1. Wash and trim the radishes. Peel the carrots and cut them into sticks.
2. In a medium bowl, combine the Greek yogurt, grated cucumber (squeeze out excess moisture), minced garlic, chopped dill, fresh lemon juice, salt, and freshly ground black pepper. Mix adequately until smooth and creamy.
3. Arrange the radish and carrot sticks on a serving platter.
4. Serve the vegetable sticks with the prepared tzatziki sauce on the side for dipping.

Nutritional Information (per serving):

- **Calories:** 70 kcal
- **Fat:** 2 g
- **Carbohydrates:** 8 g
- **Protein:** 6 g
- **Cholesterol:** 3 mg

Sliced Bell Peppers with Tuna Salad

Prep Time: 15 minutes | **Cook Time:** 0 minutes | **Servings:** 4 servings

Ingredients:

- 2 cans (5 oz each) tuna in water, drained
- 1/2 cup plain Greek yogurt
- 1 tablespoon lemon juice
- 1/2 teaspoon Dijon mustard
- 1/4 teaspoon garlic powder
- Salt and freshly ground black pepper, to taste
- 2 large bell peppers (any color), sliced into strips
- 1/4 cup chopped celery
- 1/4 cup chopped red onion
- 1 tablespoon chopped fresh parsley

Instructions:

1. In a medium bowl, combine the drained tuna, plain Greek yogurt, lemon juice, Dijon mustard, garlic powder, salt, and freshly ground black pepper. Mix adequately until all ingredients are incorporated.

2. Arrange the bell pepper slices on a serving platter.

3. Spoon the prepared tuna salad onto each bell pepper slice.

4. Top each tuna salad-filled bell pepper slice with chopped celery, chopped red onion, and fresh parsley.

Nutritional Information (per serving):

- **Calories:** 130 kcal
- **Fat:** 2 g
- **Carbohydrates:** 8 g
- **Protein:** 20 g
- **Cholesterol:** 25 mg

Chapter 7: High-Fiber Sides

Quinoa and Black Bean Salad

Prep Time: 15 minutes | **Cook Time:** 20 minutes | **Servings:** 4

Ingredients:

- 1 cup quinoa, rinsed
- 2 cups water or vegetable broth
- 1 can (15 oz) black beans, drained and rinsed
- 1 red bell pepper, diced
- 1 cup cherry tomatoes, halved
- 1/2 cup red onion, finely chopped
- 1/4 cup fresh cilantro, chopped
- 1 avocado, diced
- Juice of 1 lime
- 2 tablespoons olive oil
- Salt and pepper to taste

Instructions:

1. In a medium saucepan, bring the water or vegetable broth to a boil. Add the quinoa, reduce heat to low, cover, and simmer for about 15-20 minutes, or until quinoa is tender and liquid is absorbed. Remove from heat and let it cool.

2. In a large bowl, combine the cooked quinoa, black beans, red bell pepper, cherry tomatoes, red onion, and cilantro.

3. In a small bowl, whisk together the lime juice, olive oil, salt, and pepper.

4. Pour the dressing over the quinoa mixture and toss gently to combine.

5. Gently fold in the diced avocado.

6. Serve immediately or chill in the refrigerator before serving.

Nutritional Information:

- **Calories:** 320 kcal
- **Fat:** 14g
- **Carbohydrates:** 42g
- **Proteins:** 10g

Roasted Brussels Sprouts with Balsamic Glaze

Prep Time: 10 minutes | **Cook Time:** 25 minutes | **Servings:** 4

Ingredients:

- 1-poundBrussels sprouts, trimmed and halved
- 2 tablespoons olive oil
- Salt and pepper to taste
- 2 tablespoons balsamic vinegar
- 1 tablespoon honey or maple syrup (optional, for sweetness)

Instructions:

1. Preheat your oven to 400°F (200°C).
2. In a large bowl, toss the Brussels sprouts with olive oil, salt, and pepper until evenly coated.
3. Spread the Brussels sprouts out in a single layer on a baking sheet.
4. Roast in the preheated oven for 20-25 minutes, shaking the pan halfway through, until the Brussels sprouts are tender and caramelized.
5. In a small saucepan, heat the balsamic vinegar over medium heat until it comes to a simmer. Reduce heat to low and simmer for 2-3 minutes until the vinegar thickens slightly. If using honey or maple syrup, stir it in until combined.
6. Drizzle the balsamic glaze over the roasted Brussels sprouts before serving.

Nutritional Information:

- **Calories:** 150 kcal
- **Fat:** 7g
- **Carbohydrates:** 19g
- **Proteins:** 5g

Cauliflower Rice with Garlic and Herbs

Prep Time: 10 minutes | **Cook Time:** 10 minutes | **Servings:** 4

Ingredients:

- 1 head cauliflower, cut into florets
- 2 tablespoons olive oil
- 3 cloves garlic, minced
- 1/4 cup fresh parsley, chopped
- Salt and pepper to taste
- Juice of 1/2 lemon (optional)

Instructions:

1. In a food processor, pulse the cauliflower florets until they resemble rice grains.
2. Heat olive oil in a large skillet over medium heat. Add minced garlic and sauté for about 1 minute, until fragrant.
3. Add the cauliflower rice to the skillet. Cook, stirring frequently, for about 5-7 minutes until the cauliflower is tender but still slightly crisp.
4. Stir in chopped parsley and season with salt and pepper to taste. If desired, squeeze lemon juice over the cauliflower rice for added freshness.
5. Remove from heat and serve hot.

Nutritional Information:

- **Calories:** 120 kcal
- **Fat:** 7g
- **Carbohydrates:** 12g
- **Proteins:** 5g

Sweet Potato and Black Bean Salad

Prep Time: 15 minutes | **Cook Time:** 25 minutes | **Servings:** 4

Ingredients:

- 2 medium sweet potatoes, peeled and diced
- 1 can (15 oz) black beans, drained and rinsed
- 1 red bell pepper, diced
- 1/4 cup red onion, finely chopped
- 1/4 cup fresh cilantro, chopped
- Juice of 1 lime
- 2 tablespoons olive oil
- 1 teaspoon ground cumin
- Salt and pepper to taste

Instructions:

1. Preheat your oven to 400°F (200°C).

2. Place diced sweet potatoes on a baking sheet. Drizzle with 1 tablespoon olive oil, sprinkle with ground cumin, salt, and pepper. Toss to coat evenly.

3. Roast sweet potatoes in the preheated oven for 20-25 minutes, stirring halfway through, until tender and lightly browned. Remove from oven and let cool slightly.

4. In a large bowl, combine roasted sweet potatoes, black beans, red bell pepper, red onion, and cilantro.

5. In a small bowl, whisk together the remaining 1 tablespoon olive oil, lime juice, salt, and pepper.

6. Pour the dressing over the salad and toss gently to combine.

7. Serve immediately or chill in the refrigerator before serving.

Nutritional Information:

- **Calories:** 280 kcal
- **Fat:** 10g
- **Carbohydrates:** 40g
- **Proteins:** 8g

Lentil and Tomato Salad

Prep Time: 10 minutes | **Cook Time:** 20 minutes | **Servings:** 4

Ingredients:

- 1 cup dry lentils, rinsed
- 2 cups water or vegetable broth
- 1 cup cherry tomatoes, halved
- 1/4 cup red onion, finely chopped
- 1/4 cup fresh parsley, chopped
- 2 tablespoons olive oil
- 2 tablespoons balsamic vinegar
- 1 clove garlic, minced
- Salt and pepper to taste

Instructions:

1. In a medium saucepan, bring water or vegetable broth to a boil. Add the rinsed lentils, reduce heat to low, cover, and simmer for 15-20 minutes, or until lentils are tender but still firm. Drain any excess liquid and let cool slightly.

2. In a large bowl, combine the cooked lentils, cherry tomatoes, red onion, and parsley.

3. In a small bowl, whisk together olive oil, balsamic vinegar, minced garlic, salt, and pepper.

4. Pour the dressing over the lentil mixture and toss gently to coat.

5. Serve immediately or chill in the refrigerator for at least 30 minutes before serving to allow flavors to meld.

Nutritional Information:

- **Calories:** 250 kcal
- **Fat:** 8g
- **Carbohydrates:** 33g
- **Proteins:** 12g

Baked Asparagus with Parmesan

Prep Time: 10 minutes | **Cook Time:** 15 minutes | **Servings:** 4

Ingredients:

- 1 bunch asparagus, tough ends trimmed
- 2 tablespoons olive oil
- 1/4 cup grated Parmesan cheese
- Salt and pepper to taste

Instructions:

1. Preheat your oven to 425°F (220°C).
2. Place the trimmed asparagus spears on a baking sheet. Drizzle with olive oil and toss to coat evenly.
3. Sprinkle grated Parmesan cheese over the asparagus. Season with salt and pepper to taste.
4. Bake in the preheated oven for 12-15 minutes, or until the asparagus is tender and the cheese is lightly browned.
5. Remove from oven and serve immediately.

Nutritional Information:

- **Calories:** 120 kcal
- **Fat:** 9g
- **Carbohydrates:** 5g
- **Proteins:** 5g

Chickpea and Spinach Salad

Prep Time: 15 minutes | **Cook Time:** 0 minutes | **Servings:** 4

Ingredients:

- 1 can (15 oz) chickpeas, drained and rinsed
- 4 cups fresh spinach leaves, chopped
- 1 cup cherry tomatoes, halved
- 1/4 cup red onion, thinly sliced
- 1/4 cup fresh parsley, chopped
- 1/4 cup feta cheese, crumbled
- 2 tablespoons olive oil
- 2 tablespoons balsamic vinegar
- Salt and pepper to taste

Instructions:

1. In a large mixing bowl, combine the chickpeas, chopped spinach, cherry tomatoes, red onion, parsley, and crumbled feta cheese.

2. Drizzle olive oil and balsamic vinegar over the salad ingredients. Toss gently to coat everything evenly. Season with salt and pepper to taste.

3. Serve immediately or refrigerate for 30 minutes to allow flavors to meld before serving.

Nutritional Information:

- **Calories:** 250 kcal
- **Fat:** 12g
- **Carbohydrates:** 28g
- **Proteins:** 10g

Roasted Carrots with Thyme

Prep Time: 10 minutes | **Cook Time:** 25 minutes | **Servings:** 4

Ingredients:

- 1-poundcarrots, peeled and sliced into sticks
- 2 tablespoons olive oil
- 1 tablespoon fresh thyme leaves
- Salt and pepper to taste

Instructions:

1. Preheat your oven to 400°F (200°C). Line a baking sheet with parchment paper or foil.
2. In a large bowl, toss the carrot sticks with olive oil, fresh thyme leaves, salt, and pepper until evenly coated.
3. Spread the seasoned carrots in a single layer on the prepared baking sheet.
4. Roast in the preheated oven for 20-25 minutes, or until the carrots are tender and lightly caramelized, stirring halfway through cooking.
5. Remove from the oven and serve hot as a side dish.

Nutritional Information:

- **Calories:** 120 kcal
- **Fat:** 7g
- **Carbohydrates:** 14g
- **Proteins:** 1g

<u>Spaghetti Squash with Marinara Sauce</u>

Prep Time: 10 minutes | **Cook Time:** 40 minutes | **Servings:** 4

Ingredients:

- 1 spaghetti squash
- 2 cups marinara sauce (store-bought or homemade)
- 2 tablespoons olive oil
- 2 cloves garlic, minced
- Salt and pepper to taste
- Fresh basil leaves, chopped (for garnish)

Instructions:

1. Preheat the oven to 400°F (200°C).
2. Cut the spaghetti squash in half lengthwise and scoop out the seeds.
3. Drizzle the cut sides with olive oil and sprinkle with salt and pepper.
4. Place the squash halves cut-side down on a baking sheet lined with parchment paper.
5. Bake for 30-40 minutes, or until the squash is tender and easily pierced with a fork.
6. Let it cool slightly, then use a fork to scrape the flesh into strands.
7. In a saucepan, heat olive oil over medium heat.
8. Add minced garlic and sauté until fragrant, about 1 minute.
9. Pour in the marinara sauce and bring to a simmer.
10. Season with salt and pepper to taste.
11. Divide the spaghetti squash strands among serving plates.
12. Spoon marinara sauce over each serving.
13. Garnish with chopped fresh basil leaves.
14. Serve hot.

Nutritional Information:

- **Calories:** 180 kcal
- **Fat:** 9g
- **Carbohydrates:** 22g
- **Proteins:** 4g

Green Bean Almondine

Prep Time: 10 minutes | **Cook Time:** 10 minutes | **Servings:** 4

Ingredients:

- 1 pound green beans, ends trimmed
- 2 tablespoons olive oil
- 1/4 cup slivered almonds
- 2 cloves garlic, minced
- Salt and pepper to taste
- 1 tablespoon lemon juice
- Fresh parsley, chopped (for garnish)

Instructions:

1. Bring a large pot of salted water to a boil.
2. Add the green beans and cook for 2-3 minutes, until crisp-tender.
3. Drain the beans and immediately transfer them to a bowl of ice water to stop the cooking process.
4. Drain again and set aside.
5. In a large skillet, heat olive oil over medium heat.
6. Add slivered almonds and toast until golden brown, stirring frequently, about 2-3 minutes.
7. Remove almonds from the skillet and set aside.
8. In the same skillet, add minced garlic and sauté for 1 minute until fragrant.
9. Add the blanched green beans to the skillet.
10. Season with salt and pepper to taste.
11. Cook for 3-4 minutes, tossing frequently, until beans are heated through and well-coated with garlic and oil.
12. Drizzle lemon juice over the green beans and toss to combine.
13. Remove from heat and transfer to a serving dish.
14. Sprinkle toasted almonds and chopped fresh parsley on top.
15. Serve immediately.

Nutritional Information:

- **Calories:** 150 kcal
- **Fat:** 10g
- **Carbohydrates:** 10g
- **Proteins:** 5g

Roasted Beet and Goat Cheese Salad

Prep Time: 15 minutes | **Cook Time:** 45 minutes | **Servings:** 4

Ingredients:

- 4 medium beets, peeled and cut into wedges
- 2 tablespoons olive oil
- Salt and pepper to taste
- 4 cups mixed greens (spinach, arugula, etc.)
- 1/2 cup crumbled goat cheese
- 1/4 cup walnuts, toasted and chopped
- Balsamic vinaigrette dressing (optional)

Instructions:

1. Preheat the oven to 400°F (200°C).
2. Place the beet wedges on a baking sheet.
3. Drizzle with olive oil and season with salt and pepper.
4. Toss to coat evenly.
5. Roast in the preheated oven for 40-45 minutes, or until tender, turning halfway through. Remove from oven and let cool slightly.
6. In a large salad bowl, arrange the mixed greens.
7. Top with roasted beet wedges.
8. Sprinkle crumbled goat cheese and toasted walnuts over the salad.
9. Drizzle with balsamic vinaigrette dressing if desired.
10. Toss gently to combine.
11. Serve immediately.

Nutritional Information:

- **Calories:** 250 kcal
- **Fat:** 15g
- **Carbohydrates:** 20g
- **Proteins:** 10g

<u>Sweet Potato Wedges with Paprika</u>

Prep Time: 10 minutes | **Cook Time:** 25 minutes | **Servings:** 4

Ingredients:

- 2 large sweet potatoes, scrubbed and cut into wedges
- 2 tablespoons olive oil
- 1 teaspoon paprika
- 1/2 teaspoon garlic powder
- Salt and pepper to taste
- Fresh parsley, chopped (for garnish, optional)

Instructions:

1. Preheat the oven to 425°F (220°C). Line a baking sheet with parchment paper or aluminum foil.

2. In a large bowl, combine sweet potato wedges, olive oil, paprika, garlic powder, salt, and pepper. Toss until the sweet potato wedges are evenly coated with the seasonings.

3. Arrange the sweet potato wedges in a single layer on the prepared baking sheet.

4. Bake in the preheated oven for 20-25 minutes, flipping halfway through, or until the sweet potatoes are tender and lightly browned.

5. Remove from the oven and let cool slightly.

6. Garnish with chopped fresh parsley if desired.

7. Serve warm.

Nutritional Information:

- **Calories:** 180 kcal
- **Fat:** 7g
- **Carbohydrates:** 27g
- **Proteins:** 2g

Kale and Apple Salad with Walnuts

Prep Time: 15 minutes | **Cook Time:** 0 minutes | **Servings:** 4

Ingredients:

- 1 bunch kale, stems removed and leaves thinly sliced
- 1 apple, cored and thinly sliced
- 1/2 cup walnuts, toasted and chopped
- 1/4 cup red onion, thinly sliced
- 1/4 cup crumbled feta cheese (optional)
- 2 tablespoons olive oil
- 1 tablespoon apple cider vinegar
- 1 tablespoon honey (optional)
- Salt and pepper to taste

Instructions:

1. In a small bowl, whisk together olive oil, apple cider vinegar, honey (if using), salt, and pepper. Set aside.
2. In a large bowl, combine kale, apple slices, walnuts, red onion, and crumbled feta cheese (if using).
3. Pour the dressing over the salad ingredients.
4. Using clean hands or tongs, toss the salad until everything is evenly coated with the dressing.
5. Divide the salad among plates or bowls.
6. Serve immediately.

Nutritional Information:

- **Calories:** 220 kcal
- **Fat:** 15g
- **Carbohydrates:** 20g
- **Proteins:** 5g

Grilled Zucchini and Bell Peppers

Prep Time: 15 minutes | **Cook Time:** 10 minutes | **Servings:** 4

Ingredients:

- 2 zucchinis, sliced lengthwise
- 2 bell peppers (any color), seeded and sliced into strips
- 2 tablespoons olive oil
- 1 teaspoon dried oregano
- 1/2 teaspoon garlic powder
- Salt and pepper to taste
- Fresh parsley, chopped (for garnish)

Instructions:

1. Preheat the grill to medium-high heat.
2. In a large bowl, toss the zucchini slices and bell pepper strips with olive oil, dried oregano, garlic powder, salt, and pepper until evenly coated.
3. Place the zucchini slices and bell pepper strips on the grill.
4. Grill for about 4-5 minutes per side, or until tender and grill marks appear.
5. Take out the grilled vegetables from the grill and transfer to a serving platter.
6. Garnish with chopped fresh parsley.
7. Serve the grilled zucchini and bell peppers hot as a side dish or as part of a main meal.

Nutritional Information:

- **Calories:** 120 kcal
- **Fat:** 7g
- **Carbohydrates:** 10g
- **Proteins:** 3g

Roasted Cauliflower with Turmeric

Prep Time: 10 minutes | **Cook Time:** 25 minutes | **Servings:** 4

Ingredients:

- 1 head cauliflower, cut into florets
- 2 tablespoons olive oil
- 1 teaspoon ground turmeric
- 1/2 teaspoon ground cumin
- 1/2 teaspoon paprika
- Salt and pepper to taste
- Fresh parsley, chopped (for garnish)

Instructions:

1. Preheat the oven to 425°F (220°C).
2. In a large bowl, toss the cauliflower florets with olive oil, ground turmeric, ground cumin, paprika, salt, and pepper until evenly coated.
3. Spread the cauliflower florets in a single layer on a baking sheet.
4. Roast for 20-25 minutes, stirring halfway through, until the cauliflower is tender and golden brown.
5. Remove from the oven and transfer to a serving dish.
6. Garnish with chopped fresh parsley.
7. Serve the roasted cauliflower with turmeric hot as a side dish or incorporate it into a main meal.

Nutritional Information:

- **Calories:** 120 kcal
- **Fat:** 7g
- **Carbohydrates:** 10g
- **Proteins:** 5g

Cabbage and Carrot Slaw with Vinegar Dressing

Prep Time: 15 minutes | **Cook Time:** 0 minutes | **Servings:** 4

Ingredients:

- 4 cups shredded cabbage
- 1 cup shredded carrots
- 2 tablespoons olive oil
- 3 tablespoons apple cider vinegar
- 1 tablespoon honey (optional, omit for lower sugar)
- Salt and pepper to taste
- Fresh parsley or cilantro, chopped (for garnish)

Instructions:

1. In a small bowl, whisk together olive oil, apple cider vinegar, honey (if using), salt, and pepper until well combined.
2. In a large bowl, combine shredded cabbage and shredded carrots.
3. Pour the dressing over the cabbage and carrots. Toss until evenly coated.
4. For enhanced flavor, refrigerate the slaw for 30 minutes before serving.
5. Garnish with chopped fresh parsley or cilantro before serving.

Nutritional Information:

- **Calories:** 120 kcal
- **Fat:** 7g
- **Carbohydrates:** 12g
- **Proteins:** 2g

Lentil and Quinoa Stuffed Tomatoes

Prep Time: 20 minutes | **Cook Time:** 30 minutes | **Servings:** 4

Ingredients:

- 4 large tomatoes
- 1/2 cup quinoa, rinsed
- 1/2 cup green or brown lentils, rinsed
- 1 cup vegetable broth
- 1 small onion, finely chopped
- 2 cloves garlic, minced
- 1 teaspoon olive oil
- 1 teaspoon dried thyme
- 1 teaspoon dried oregano
- Salt and pepper to taste
- Fresh parsley or basil, chopped (for garnish)

Instructions:

1. Preheat the oven to 375°F (190°C).
2. Slice off the tops of the tomatoes and carefully scoop out the seeds and pulp to create a hollow cavity. Set aside.
3. In a medium saucepan, heat olive oil over medium heat. Add chopped onion and garlic, sauté until translucent.
4. Add quinoa, lentils, vegetable broth, dried thyme, dried oregano, salt, and pepper. Bring to a boil.
5. Reduce heat, cover, and simmer for 15-20 minutes, or until quinoa and lentils are tender and liquid is absorbed. Remove from heat.
6. Spoon the quinoa and lentil mixture evenly into the hollowed-out tomatoes.
7. Place stuffed tomatoes in a baking dish. Cover loosely with foil.
8. Bake for 20-25 minutes, or until tomatoes are tender and heated through.
9. Garnish with chopped fresh parsley or basil before serving.

Nutritional Information:

- **Calories:** 220 kcal
- **Fat:** 3g
- **Carbohydrates:** 38g
- **Proteins:** 11g

Steamed Broccoli with Lemon Zest

Prep Time: 10 minutes | **Cook Time:** 10 minutes | **Servings:** 4

Ingredients:

- 1-pound(450g) broccoli florets
- Zest of 1 lemon
- 1 tablespoon olive oil
- Salt and pepper to taste
- Lemon wedges (for serving)

Instructions:

1. Cut broccoli into florets, ensuring they are bite-sized.
2. Fill a steamer pot with water just below the steamer basket. Bring the water to a boil.
3. Place broccoli florets in the steamer basket. Cover and steam for 5-7 minutes, or until broccoli is tender-crisp.
4. In a small bowl, combine olive oil and lemon zest.
5. Transfer steamed broccoli to a serving dish.
6. Drizzle with lemon zest and olive oil mixture. Season with salt and pepper to taste.
7. Serve hot with lemon wedges on the side.

Nutritional Information:

- **Calories:** 70 kcal
- **Fat:** 4g
- **Carbohydrates:** 8g
- **Proteins:** 3g

Sautéed Spinach with Garlic

Prep Time: 5 minutes | **Cook Time:** 5 minutes | **Servings:** 4

Ingredients:

- 1-pound(450g) fresh spinach leaves, washed and stemmed
- 3 cloves garlic, minced
- 1 tablespoon olive oil
- Salt and pepper to taste

Instructions:

1. Wash the spinach thoroughly and remove any tough stems.
2. In a large skillet, heat olive oil over medium heat.
3. Add minced garlic to the skillet and sauté for about 1 minute until fragrant.
4. Add the spinach to the skillet in batches, stirring constantly until wilted. Cook for about 3-4 minutes until spinach is tender.
5. Season with salt and pepper to taste.
6. Remove from heat and transfer to a serving dish.

Nutritional Information:

- **Calories:** 60 kcal
- **Fat:** 4g
- **Carbohydrates:** 5g
- **Proteins:** 3g

Chapter 8: Nutrient-Dense Desserts

Chia Seed Pudding with Coconut Milk

Prep Time: 10 minutes | **Cook Time:** 0 minutes | **Servings:** 4

Ingredients:

- 1/2 cup chia seeds
- 2 cups unsweetened coconut milk
- 1 teaspoon vanilla extract
- 2 tablespoons maple syrup (optional, adjust to taste)
- Fresh berries, for topping
- Unsweetened shredded coconut, for topping

Instructions:

1. In a mixing bowl, combine chia seeds, coconut milk, vanilla extract, and maple syrup (if using). Stir adequately to combine.
2. Cover the bowl and refrigerate for at least 2 hours or overnight, stirring occasionally, until the mixture thickens and the chia seeds have absorbed the liquid.
3. Once thickened, stir the pudding to redistribute the chia seeds evenly.
4. Serve chilled, topped with fresh berries and shredded coconut.

Nutritional Information:

- **Calories:** 180 kcal
- **Fat:** 12g
- **Carbohydrates:** 14g
- **Proteins:** 5g

Avocado Chocolate Mousse

Prep Time: 10 minutes | **Cook Time:** 0 minutes | **Servings:** 4

Ingredients:

- 2 ripe avocados, peeled and pitted
- 1/4 cup unsweetened cocoa powder
- 1/4 cup coconut milk
- 1/4 cup maple syrup or honey (adjust to taste)
- 1 teaspoon vanilla extract
- Fresh berries, for garnish (optional)

Instructions:

1. In a food processor or blender, combine the avocados, cocoa powder, coconut milk, maple syrup (or honey), and vanilla extract.
2. Blend until smooth and creamy, scraping down the sides as needed to ensure everything is well mixed.
3. Divide the mousse into serving dishes and refrigerate for at least 1 hour to chill and set.
4. Serve chilled, garnished with fresh berries if desired.

Nutritional Information:

- **Calories:** 190 kcal
- **Fat:** 12g
- **Carbohydrates:** 20g
- **Proteins:** 3g

Almond Flour Brownies

Prep Time: 15 minutes | **Cook Time:** 25 minutes | **Servings:** 12

Ingredients:

- 1 cup almond flour
- 1/4 cup unsweetened cocoa powder
- 1/2 teaspoon baking soda
- 1/4 teaspoon salt
- 1/4 cup coconut oil, melted
- 1/2 cup maple syrup or honey
- 2 large eggs
- 1 teaspoon vanilla extract
- 1/2 cup dark chocolate chips (optional)
- Chopped nuts, for topping (optional)

Instructions:

1. Preheat the oven to 350°F (175°C). Grease or line an 8x8 inch baking pan with parchment paper.
2. In a mixing bowl, whisk together almond flour, cocoa powder, baking soda, and salt.
3. In another bowl, whisk together melted coconut oil, maple syrup (or honey), eggs, and vanilla extract until well combined.
4. Add the wet ingredients to the dry ingredients and stir until smooth.
5. Fold in dark chocolate chips if using.
6. Pour the batter into the prepared baking pan and spread evenly.
7. Bake for 20-25 minutes, or until a toothpick inserted into the center comes out mostly clean with a few crumbs attached.
8. Remove from the oven and let cool completely in the pan on a wire rack.
9. Once cooled, slice into squares and top with chopped nuts if desired.

Nutritional Information:

- **Calories:** 180 kcal
- **Fat:** 12g
- **Carbohydrates:** 16g
- **Proteins:** 4g

Coconut Macaroons

Prep Time: 10 minutes | **Cook Time:** 20 minutes | **Servings:** 12

Ingredients:

- 3 cups shredded coconut, unsweetened
- 1/2 cup almond flour
- 1/2 cup maple syrup or honey
- 1/4 cup coconut oil, melted
- 1 teaspoon vanilla extract
- 1/4 teaspoon salt
- 2 large egg whites

Instructions:

1. Preheat the oven to 325°F (160°C). Line a baking sheet with parchment paper.
2. In a large bowl, combine shredded coconut, almond flour, maple syrup (or honey), melted coconut oil, vanilla extract, and salt. Mix adequately.
3. In a separate bowl, beat the egg whites until stiff peaks form.
4. Gently fold the beaten egg whites into the coconut mixture until thoroughly combined.
5. Using a spoon or cookie scoop, drop rounded tablespoons of the mixture onto the prepared baking sheet, spacing them about 1 inch apart.
6. Bake for 18-20 minutes, or until the edges are golden brown.
7. Remove from the oven and let cool on the baking sheet for 5 minutes, then transfer to a wire rack to cool completely.

Nutritional Information:

- **Calories:** 180 kcal
- **Fat:** 12g
- **Carbohydrates:** 15g
- **Proteins:** 2g

Berry and Greek Yogurt Parfait

Prep Time: 10 minutes | **Cook Time:** 0 minutes | **Servings:** 2

Ingredients:

- 1 cup plain Greek yogurt
- 1 cup mixed berries (such as strawberries, blueberries, raspberries)
- 2 tablespoons unsweetened shredded coconut
- 2 tablespoons chopped nuts (such as almonds or walnuts)
- 1 tablespoon honey or maple syrup (optional)

Instructions:

1. In two serving glasses or bowls, layer half of the Greek yogurt.
2. Top with half of the mixed berries, shredded coconut, and chopped nuts.
3. Drizzle with honey or maple syrup if using.
4. Repeat the layers with the remaining Greek yogurt, berries, coconut, and nuts.
5. Serve immediately or refrigerate until ready to serve.

Nutritional Information:

- **Calories:** 220 kcal
- **Fat:** 10g
- **Carbohydrates:** 22g
- **Proteins:** 12g

Dark Chocolate and Nut Clusters

Prep Time: 10 minutes | **Cook Time:** 5 minutes | **Servings:** 12 clusters

Ingredients:

- 1 cup mixed nuts (such as almonds, walnuts, pecans), chopped
- 1/2 cup dark chocolate chips (at least 70% cocoa)
- 1 tablespoon coconut oil
- 1/4 teaspoon vanilla extract
- Pinch of sea salt

Instructions:

1. Line a baking sheet with parchment paper.
2. In a microwave-safe bowl or using a double boiler, melt the dark chocolate chips and coconut oil together until smooth.
3. Stir in the vanilla extract and a pinch of sea salt.
4. Add the chopped mixed nuts to the melted chocolate mixture and stir until well combined.
5. Spoon tablespoon-sized clusters onto the prepared baking sheet.
6. Refrigerate for about 30 minutes, or until the chocolate has set.
7. Once set, store the clusters in an airtight container in the refrigerator.

Nutritional Information:

- **Calories:** 120 kcal
- **Fat:** 9g
- **Carbohydrates:** 7g
- **Proteins:** 3g

Almond Butter and Banana Bites

Prep Time: 10 minutes | **Cook Time:** 0 minutes | **Servings:** 12 bites

Ingredients:

- 2 ripe bananas
- 1/2 cup almond butter
- 1/4 cup unsweetened shredded coconut
- 1/4 cup chopped almonds
- 1 tablespoon chia seeds
- 1/2 teaspoon ground cinnamon

Instructions:

1. Peel the bananas and cut them into slices.
2. Spread almond butter on one side of each banana slice.
3. In a small bowl, mix together shredded coconut, chopped almonds, chia seeds, and ground cinnamon.
4. Dip each almond butter-coated banana slice into the coconut mixture, pressing gently to coat.
5. Place the coated banana slices on a plate or baking sheet lined with parchment paper.
6. Refrigerate for about 30 minutes to allow the bites to set.
7. Once set, store in an airtight container in the refrigerator.

Nutritional Information:

- **Calories:** 110 kcal
- **Fat:** 7g
- **Carbohydrates:** 10g
- **Proteins:** 3g

Coconut Flour Banana Bread

Prep Time: 15 minutes | **Cook Time:** 45 minutes | **Servings:** 12 slices

Ingredients:

- 4 medium ripe bananas
- 4 large eggs
- 1/2 cup coconut flour
- 1/4 cup coconut oil, melted
- 1/4 cup honey or maple syrup (optional, omit for lower sugar content)
- 1 teaspoon vanilla extract
- 1 teaspoon baking soda
- 1/2 teaspoon ground cinnamon
- 1/4 teaspoon salt

Instructions:

1. Preheat your oven to 350°F (175°C). Grease a 9x5 inch loaf pan or line it with parchment paper.

2. In a large mixing bowl, mash the bananas until smooth.

3. Add the eggs, melted coconut oil, honey or maple syrup (if using), and vanilla extract to the mashed bananas. Mix adequately until combined.

4. In a separate bowl, whisk together the coconut flour, baking soda, cinnamon, and salt.

5. Gradually add the dry ingredients to the wet ingredients, mixing until smooth and well combined.

6. Pour the batter into the prepared loaf pan, spreading it evenly.

7. Bake for 40-45 minutes, or until the top is golden brown and a toothpick inserted into the center comes out clean.

8. Allow the banana bread to cool in the pan for 10 minutes, then transfer it to a wire rack to cool completely before slicing.

Nutritional Information:

- **Calories:** 150 kcal
- **Fat:** 8g
- **Carbohydrates:** 16g
- **Proteins:** 4g

Blueberry and Almond Chia Pudding

Prep Time: 10 minutes | **Cook Time:** 0 minutes | **Servings:** 2

Ingredients:

- 1/2 cup chia seeds
- 1 1/2 cups unsweetened almond milk
- 1/2 teaspoon vanilla extract
- 1 tablespoon honey or maple syrup (optional, omit for lower sugar content)
- 1/2 cup fresh blueberries
- 2 tablespoons sliced almonds

Instructions:

1. In a mixing bowl, combine the chia seeds, almond milk, vanilla extract, and honey or maple syrup (if using). Stir adequately until all ingredients are thoroughly mixed.

2. Let the mixture sit for 5 minutes, then stir again to prevent clumping. Cover the bowl and refrigerate for at least 2 hours, or preferably overnight, to allow the chia seeds to absorb the liquid and thicken.

3. Once the chia pudding has thickened to your desired consistency, divide it into serving bowls or jars.

4. Top each serving with fresh blueberries and sliced almonds.

5. Serve chilled and enjoy!

Nutritional Information:

- **Calories:** 250 kcal
- **Fat:** 15g
- **Carbohydrates:** 25g
- **Proteins:** 8g

Baked Apple with Cinnamon and Walnuts

Prep Time: 10 minutes | **Cook Time:** 30 minutes | **Servings:** 2

Ingredients:

- 2 medium apples (such as Granny Smith or Honeycrisp)
- 1/4 teaspoon ground cinnamon
- 2 tablespoons chopped walnuts
- 1 tablespoon honey or maple syrup (optional, omit for lower sugar content)
- 1/4 cup water

Instructions:

1. Preheat the oven to 375°F (190°C).
2. Core the apples using an apple corer or a small knife, leaving the bottoms intact.
3. Place the apples in a baking dish. Sprinkle each apple with half of the cinnamon and fill the centers with chopped walnuts. Drizzle with honey or maple syrup if using.
4. Pour water into the bottom of the baking dish around the apples.
5. Cover the baking dish with foil and bake for 20 minutes. Take out the foil and bake for an additional 10 minutes or until the apples are tender.
6. Remove from the oven and let cool slightly before serving.

Nutritional Information:

- **Calories:** 180 kcal
- **Fat:** 6g
- **Carbohydrates:** 32g
- **Proteins:** 2g

Dark Chocolate Avocado Truffles

Prep Time: 15 minutes | **Cook Time:** 0 minutes | **Servings:** 12 truffles

Ingredients:

- 1 ripe avocado, mashed
- 100g dark chocolate (70% cocoa or higher), melted
- 2 tablespoons cocoa powder
- 1/2 teaspoon vanilla extract
- Pinch of salt
- Optional toppings: unsweetened shredded coconut, chopped nuts, cocoa powder

Instructions:

1. In a mixing bowl, combine the mashed avocado, melted dark chocolate, cocoa powder, vanilla extract, and salt until smooth and well blended.
2. Place the mixture in the refrigerator for about 10-15 minutes to firm up slightly.
3. Once the mixture is firm enough to handle, scoop out tablespoon-sized portions and roll into balls.
4. Roll each truffle in your choice of optional toppings like unsweetened shredded coconut, chopped nuts, or cocoa powder.
5. Place the truffles on a plate or baking sheet lined with parchment paper.
6. Refrigerate the truffles for at least 30 minutes to allow them to set.
7. Serve chilled. Store any leftovers in an airtight container in the refrigerator.

Nutritional Information:

- **Calories:** 70 kcal
- **Fat:** 5g
- **Carbohydrates:** 5g
- **Proteins:** 1g

Lemon and Almond Flour Cookies

Prep Time: 15 minutes | **Cook Time:** 12 minutes | **Servings:** 12 cookies

Ingredients:

- 1 cup almond flour
- 1/4 cup coconut flour
- 1/4 teaspoon baking soda
- Pinch of salt
- Zest of 1 lemon
- 2 tablespoons fresh lemon juice
- 1/4 cup honey or maple syrup (adjust according to sweetness preference)
- 1/4 cup coconut oil, melted
- 1 teaspoon vanilla extract

Instructions:

1. Preheat the oven to 350°F (175°C) and line a baking sheet with parchment paper.

2. In a mixing bowl, whisk together almond flour, coconut flour, baking soda, salt, and lemon zest.

3. In a separate bowl, mix together lemon juice, honey or maple syrup, melted coconut oil, and vanilla extract.

4. Pour the wet ingredients into the dry ingredients and stir until well combined and a dough forms.

5. Scoop tablespoon-sized portions of dough and roll them into balls. Place them on the prepared baking sheet.

6. Use a fork to gently flatten each ball into a cookie shape.

7. Bake for 10-12 minutes, or until the edges are golden brown.

8. Remove from the oven and let the cookies cool on the baking sheet for 5 minutes before transferring them to a wire rack to cool completely.

Nutritional Information:

- **Calories:** 110 kcal
- **Fat:** 8g
- **Carbohydrates:** 8g
- **Proteins:** 2g

Raspberry and Coconut Bars

Prep Time: 15 minutes | **Cook Time:** 25 minutes | **Number of Servings:** 12 bars

Ingredients:

- 1 cup almond flour
- 1/4 cup coconut flour
- 1/4 teaspoon baking soda
- Pinch of salt
- 1/4 cup coconut oil, melted
- 1/4 cup honey or maple syrup (adjust according to sweetness preference)
- 1 teaspoon vanilla extract
- 1 cup fresh raspberries
- 1/2 cup unsweetened shredded coconut

Instructions:

1. Preheat the oven to 350°F (175°C). Line an 8x8-inch baking dish with parchment paper, leaving some overhang for easy removal later.

2. In a large mixing bowl, combine almond flour, coconut flour, baking soda, and salt.

3. In a separate bowl, whisk together melted coconut oil, honey or maple syrup, and vanilla extract.

4. Pour the wet ingredients into the dry ingredients and mix until well combined and a dough forms.

5. Press about two-thirds of the dough evenly into the bottom of the prepared baking dish to form the crust.

6. Evenly distribute the raspberries over the crust, gently pressing them into the dough.

7. Sprinkle the shredded coconut over the raspberries.

8. Crumble the remaining dough evenly over the top as a crumble topping.

9. Bake for 20-25 minutes, or until the top is lightly golden brown.

10. Remove from the oven and let cool completely in the pan on a wire rack.

11. Once cooled, lift the bars out of the pan using the parchment paper overhang and cut into squares or bars.

Nutritional Information:

- **Calories:** 160 kcal
- **Fat:** 10g
- **Carbohydrates:** 14g
- **Proteins:** 2g

Pumpkin and Almond Butter Cookies

Prep Time: 15 minutes | **Cook Time:** 12 minutes | **Number of Servings:** 12 cookies

Ingredients:

- 1 cup almond flour
- 1/2 cup canned pumpkin puree
- 1/4 cup almond butter
- 1/4 cup honey or maple syrup
- 1 teaspoon vanilla extract
- 1 teaspoon ground cinnamon
- 1/4 teaspoon ground nutmeg
- 1/4 teaspoon baking soda
- Pinch of salt
- 1/4 cup chopped walnuts (optional)

Instructions:

1. Preheat the oven to 350°F (175°C). Line a baking sheet with parchment paper.
2. In a large mixing bowl, combine almond flour, pumpkin puree, almond butter, honey or maple syrup, vanilla extract, cinnamon, nutmeg, baking soda, and salt. Mix until well combined.
3. If using, fold in chopped walnuts into the dough.
4. Scoop about 1.5 tablespoons of dough per cookie and place onto the prepared baking sheet, leaving space between each cookie.
5. Flatten each cookie slightly with the back of a spoon or fork.
6. Bake for 10-12 minutes, or until edges are golden brown.
7. Remove from the oven and let the cookies cool on the baking sheet for 5 minutes, then transfer them to a wire rack to cool completely.

Nutritional Information:

- **Calories:** 140 kcal
- **Fat:** 9g
- **Carbohydrates:** 11g
- **Proteins:** 4g

Strawberry and Chia Seed Jam Bars

Prep Time: 15 minutes | **Cook Time:** 30 minutes | **Number of Servings:** 12 bars

Ingredients:

- 2 cups almond flour
- 1/4 cup coconut oil, melted
- 1/4 cup honey or maple syrup
- 1 teaspoon vanilla extract
- 1/4 teaspoon salt
- 1 cup fresh strawberries, diced
- 2 tablespoons chia seeds
- 1 tablespoon lemon juice
- 2 tablespoons water
- 1 tablespoon honey or maple syrup (optional, for additional sweetness)

Instructions:

1. Preheat the oven to 350°F (175°C). Line an 8x8-inch baking pan with parchment paper.

2. In a mixing bowl, combine almond flour, melted coconut oil, honey or maple syrup, vanilla extract, and salt. Mix until crumbly.

3. Reserve 3/4 cup of the mixture for topping and press the rest evenly into the bottom of the prepared baking pan.

4. In a saucepan, combine diced strawberries, chia seeds, lemon juice, water, and optional honey or maple syrup. Bring to a simmer over medium heat, stirring occasionally, until thickened (about 5-7 minutes).

5. Take out the strawberry mixture from heat and let it cool slightly.

6. Pour the strawberry jam over the crust in the baking pan, spreading evenly.

7. Sprinkle the reserved almond flour mixture evenly over the top of the strawberry jam.

8. Bake in the preheated oven for 25-30 minutes, or until the top is lightly golden brown.

9. Remove from the oven and let cool completely in the pan on a wire rack.

10. Once cooled, lift the bars out of the pan using the parchment paper, then cut into 12 bars.

Nutritional Information:

- **Calories:** 180 kcal
- **Fat:** 12g
- **Carbohydrates:** 15g
- **Proteins:** 4g

Low-Sugar Chocolate Chip Cookies

Prep Time: 15 minutes | **Cook Time:** 10 minutes | **Number of Servings:** 24 cookies

Ingredients:

- 1/2 cup almond flour
- 1/4 cup coconut flour
- 1/2 teaspoon baking soda
- 1/4 teaspoon salt
- 1/4 cup coconut oil, melted
- 1/4 cup honey or maple syrup
- 1 large egg
- 1 teaspoon vanilla extract
- 1/2 cup dark chocolate chips (sugar-free or stevia-sweetened preferred)

Instructions:

1. Preheat the oven to 350°F (175°C). Line a baking sheet with parchment paper.
2. In a mixing bowl, whisk together almond flour, coconut flour, baking soda, and salt.
3. In a separate bowl, mix melted coconut oil and honey (or maple syrup) until well combined.
4. Add the egg and vanilla extract to the wet ingredients, stirring until smooth.
5. Gradually add the dry ingredients to the wet ingredients, mixing until a dough forms.
6. Fold in the dark chocolate chips.
7. Drop rounded tablespoons of dough onto the prepared baking sheet, spacing them about 2 inches apart.
8. Flatten each cookie slightly with the back of a spoon or your fingers.
9. Bake for 8-10 minutes, or until the edges are golden brown.
10. Remove from the oven and let the cookies cool on the baking sheet for 5 minutes, then transfer to a wire rack to cool completely.

Nutritional Information:

- **Calories:** 90 kcal
- **Fat:** 6g
- **Carbohydrates:** 8g
- **Proteins:** 2g

Coconut and Lime Energy Balls

Prep Time: 15 minutes | **Cook Time:** No cook | **Number of Servings:** 12 balls

Ingredients:

- 1 cup shredded Coconut (unsweetened)
- 1 cup Almonds
- 10 Medjool Dates, pitted
- Zest and juice of 2 Limes
- 2 tablespoons Chia Seeds
- 1 tablespoon Coconut Oil
- Pinch of Salt

Instructions:

1. In a food processor, combine shredded Coconut and Almonds. Pulse until finely ground.
2. Add pitted Dates, Lime zest and juice, Chia Seeds, Coconut Oil, and Salt. Process until the mixture comes together and becomes sticky.
3. Roll the mixture into 12 balls, about 1 tablespoon each.
4. Place the balls on a baking sheet lined with parchment paper and refrigerate for at least 30 minutes before serving.

Nutritional Information:

- **Cal:** 120 kcal
- **Fat:** 8 g
- **Carbs:** 11 g
- **Proteins:** 2 g

Dark Chocolate and Almond Butter Cups

Prep Time: 15 minutes | **Cook Time:** No cook | **Number of Servings:** 12 cups

Ingredients:

- 1 cup Dark Chocolate Chips (at least 70% cocoa)
- 1/2 cup Almond Butter (unsweetened)
- 1 tablespoon Coconut Oil
- 1/4 teaspoon Vanilla Extract
- Sea Salt, to sprinkle on top (optional)

Instructions:

1. Line a mini muffin tin with 12 paper or silicone liners.
2. In a microwave-safe bowl, combine Dark Chocolate Chips and Coconut Oil. Microwave in 30-second intervals, stirring in between, until completely melted and smooth.
3. Spoon 1 teaspoon of melted Chocolate into each liner, spreading it halfway up the sides.
4. In another bowl, mix Almond Butter and Vanilla Extract until smooth. Place a small amount (about 1 teaspoon) of Almond Butter mixture into each chocolate-lined cup.
5. Cover each cup with remaining melted Chocolate, ensuring the Almond Butter is completely covered.
6. Sprinkle Sea Salt on top if desired.
7. Refrigerate for at least 1 hour until set.
8. Once set, take out the paper or silicone liners and store in an airtight container in the refrigerator.

Nutritional Information:

- **Cal:** 140 kcal
- **Fat:** 11 g
- **Carbs:** 8 g
- **Proteins:** 3 g

<u>Baked Pear with Honey and Almonds</u>

Prep Time: 10 minutes | **Cook Time:** 25 minutes | **Number of Servings:** 4

Ingredients:

- 4 Pears, ripe but firm

- 2 tablespoons Honey

- 1/4 cup Almonds, chopped

- 1/2 teaspoon Cinnamon

- 1 tablespoon Butter, melted

Instructions:

1. Preheat the oven to 375°F (190°C).

2. Wash and dry the pears. Cut each pear in half lengthwise and core them, creating a hollow in the center.

3. Place the pear halves cut side up in a baking dish.

4. In a small bowl, mix together the chopped almonds, cinnamon, and melted butter.

5. Spoon the almond mixture into the hollow of each pear half.

6. Drizzle honey evenly over the pears.

7. Cover the baking dish with foil and bake for 20 minutes.

8. Take out the foil and bake for an additional 5-7 minutes, or until the pears are tender and the almonds are lightly toasted.

9. Serve warm, optionally with a dollop of Greek yogurt or a sprinkle of additional cinnamon.

Nutritional Information:

- **Cal:** 190 kcal

- **Fat:** 7 g

- **Carbs:** 34 g

- **Proteins:** 2 g

Cinnamon and Flaxseed Muffins

Prep Time: 15 minutes | **Cook Time:** 20 minutes | **Number of Servings:** 12

Ingredients:

- 2 cups Almond Flour
- 1/2 cup Ground Flaxseed
- 1/4 cup Coconut Flour
- 2 teaspoons Baking Powder
- 1/2 teaspoon Baking Soda
- 1/2 teaspoon Salt
- 2 teaspoons Cinnamon
- 4 large Eggs
- 1/4 cup Coconut Oil, melted
- 1/3 cup Unsweetened Applesauce
- 1/3 cup Honey or Maple Syrup
- 1 teaspoon Vanilla Extract

Instructions:

1. Preheat the oven to 350°F (175°C). Line a muffin tin with paper liners or grease well.

2. In a large bowl, combine almond flour, ground flaxseed, coconut flour, baking powder, baking soda, salt, and cinnamon.

3. In another bowl, whisk together eggs, melted coconut oil, applesauce, honey or maple syrup, and vanilla extract.

4. Pour the wet ingredients into the dry ingredients and stir until well combined and no lumps remain.

5. Divide the batter evenly among the muffin cups, filling each about 2/3 full.

6. Bake for 18-20 minutes, or until a toothpick inserted into the center comes out clean.

7. Remove from the oven and let the muffins cool in the tin for 5 minutes, then transfer them to a wire rack to cool completely.

Nutritional Information:

- **Cal:** 180 kcal
- **Fat:** 14 g
- **Carbs:** 10 g
- **Proteins:** 6 g

Chapter 9

Lifestyle and Practical Tips

Meal Planning and Preparation

Effectively adhering to the Galveston Diet requires careful consideration of meal planning and preparation to maintain progress toward your nutritional objectives. Here are some valuable tips to help you make this process more efficient:

1. Weekly Meal Planning:

- **Set Aside Time:** Set aside a dedicated time each week to plan your meals. This helps prevent making impulsive food choices that may not align with your dietary preferences.

- **Create a Menu:** Plan breakfast, lunch, dinner, and snacks for the entire week. Incorporate a balanced combination of healthy fats, lean proteins, and fiber-rich carbohydrates into every meal.

- **Balanced Meals:** Strive for a well-balanced plate during each meal. For instance, a dinner could consist of grilled salmon (a good source of protein and healthy fat), a side of quinoa (a fiber-rich carbohydrate), and steamed broccoli (a serving of vegetables).

2. Efficient Grocery Shopping:

- **Create a List:** Write a detailed grocery list according to your meal plan. Stick to the list to avoid making impulsive purchases that can derail your diet.

- **Shop the Perimeter:** Shop the perimeter of the grocery store, as that's where you'll find most of the whole, unprocessed foods. Direct your shopping to this location to find fresh produce, lean proteins, and healthy fats.

- **Buy in Bulk:** Consider buying staple items like nuts, seeds, and whole grains in bulk to save money and reduce the frequency of shopping trips.

3. Food Preparation:

- **Batch Cooking:** Prepare generous portions of meals and divide them into smaller servings for the week. This can involve cooking grains, roasting vegetables, and grilling proteins.

- **Use Containers:** Consider investing in durable, reusable containers for storing your pre-prepared meals. Transparent containers provide a convenient way to view the contents.

- **Prepare Ingredients:** Ensure that vegetables are thoroughly washed and chopped, proteins are marinated, and snacks are portioned ahead of time. This simplifies putting together meals efficiently on hectic days.

Intermittent Fasting

Intermittent fasting (IF) is essential to the Galveston Diet, providing various health benefits, including boosted metabolism, improved cellular repair, and increased insulin sensitivity. Here's a simple guide to integrating intermittent fasting into your daily routine:

1. Understanding Fasting Windows:

- **16/8 Method:** The 16/8 Method involves fasting for 16 hours and consuming all meals within an 8-hour window. As an illustration, you could consider finishing your meal at 8 PM and having your first meal at noon the following day.

- **14/10 Method:** Try fasting for 14 hours and eating within a 10-hour window using the 14/10 method. This could be helpful for beginners who initially struggle with the 16/8 method.

- **5:2 Method:** The 5:2 Method involves eating normally for five days a week and then restricting calorie intake to 500-600 calories on two non-consecutive days.

2. Tips for Success:

- **Stay Hydrated:** Remember to drink plenty of water, herbal teas, and black coffee during fasting periods. This will help keep you hydrated and reduce feelings of hunger.

- **Listen to Your Body:** Listen to your body's signals. If you experience dizziness or excessive hunger, adjust your fasting window or method. It's crucial to discover a routine that suits your needs.

- **Gradual Transition:** Begin with a shorter fasting period and slowly extend the fasting window as your body becomes accustomed to it.

3. Benefits of Intermittent Fasting:

- **Improved Metabolism:** Fasting can boost your metabolic rate, increasing calorie burning.

- **Cellular Repair:** Fasting can trigger a process called autophagy, which helps cells remove and repair damaged components.

- **Improved Insulin Sensitivity:** Reduced eating windows have been shown to positively impact insulin levels, leading to better blood sugar control and a decreased risk of type 2 diabetes.

Exercise and Managing Stress

It is essential to incorporate regular physical activity and effective stress management techniques alongside your dietary changes to promote overall well-being. Here's a guide on incorporating these practices into your daily routine:

1. Physical Activity:

- **Regular Exercise:** Aim for at least 150 minutes of moderate-intensity aerobic activity or 75 minutes of vigorous-intensity activity each week. Additionally, don't forget to incorporate muscle-strengthening activities on two or more days.

- **Variety of Exercises:** Include a wide range of exercises to target different aspects of fitness. This can be a mix of cardio (walking, jogging, cycling), strength training (weight lifting, resistance bands), and flexibility exercises (yoga, stretching).

- **Consistency:** Consistency is key to sticking with your exercise routine. Find activities you genuinely enjoy, as this will make it easier for you to stay motivated and committed. By doing so, you'll be able to maintain a regular exercise schedule and reap the benefits of a healthy and active lifestyle. Consistency is critical for maximizing the benefits of regular physical activity.

2. Stress Management Techniques:

- **Mindfulness and Meditation:** Incorporate mindfulness practices like meditation, deep breathing exercises, or yoga into your routine. These practices can help reduce stress and improve mental clarity.

- **Adequate Sleep:** To maintain a healthy sleep routine, ensure you get 7-9 hours of quality sleep each night. Inadequate sleep can increase stress levels and have detrimental effects on your health.

- **Leisure Activities:** Every once in a while, engage in activities that bring you joy and help you unwind, such as reading, gardening, or spending quality time with loved ones. Carving out time for hobbies can remarkably impact reducing stress levels.

3. Benefits of Exercise and Stress Management:

- **Enhanced Mood:** Regular physical activity and stress management have been shown to have a positive impact on mood and can help reduce symptoms of anxiety and depression.

- **Better Physical Health:** Exercise has numerous benefits for your physical health. It can improve the strength of your heart, muscles, and bones, which can help reduce the risk of chronic diseases. Additionally, effective stress management techniques can also contribute to better overall health.

- **Enhanced Focus and Productivity:** Reducing stress and sticking to a consistent exercise routine can improve cognitive function and overall productivity.

By incorporating these practical tips for meal planning, intermittent fasting, and lifestyle adjustments, you can wholeheartedly embrace the Galveston Diet and experience long-term health benefits. This comprehensive approach guarantees that you not only achieve your nutritional objectives but also promote your overall physical and mental health.

Conclusion

Embarking on the journey with the Galveston diet involves more than just modifying your diet. It's a holistic approach that aims to transform your lifestyle for long-term health and vitality. As you've explored the principles of this diet, delved into nutritious meal planning, understood the benefits of intermittent fasting, and embraced the importance of exercise and stress management, you've gained valuable knowledge to improve your overall health.

This cookbook is a valuable resource for making sustainable, positive changes that perfectly align with your body's needs. By prioritizing whole, nutrient-dense foods and maintaining a balanced approach to eating, you are making progress toward your weight loss goals, promoting hormonal balance, and decreasing inflammation. Remember, the Galveston Diet is a flexible and adaptable plan designed to fit seamlessly into your life.

As you explore the mouthwatering recipes and practical tips provided, you'll experience a renewed sense of health and vitality. Stay dedicated to this journey, pay attention to your body, and make any necessary changes to ensure that this diet becomes a long-term part of your lifestyle.

Thank you for choosing to embark on this path with the "*Galveston Diet Cookbook for Beginners*." Cheers to a healthier, happier you! Embrace the journey, relish the delicious flavors, and celebrate your milestones every step of the way.

Recipes Index